Advance Praise for *Exposure Therapy for Eating Disorders*

"This book expertly and informatively explains the why and how of exposure for eating disorders and its essential role across different treatment modalities. A must-read for all those therapists who anxiously wonder 'what if my client falls apart if I get them to face what they avoid.'"
—**Tracey Wade,** PhD, Matthew Flinders Distinguished Professor, Flinders University

"A comprehensive understanding of exposure-based principles and techniques is essential for all clinicians working in the treatment of eating disorders. This book is a masterpiece in which three brilliant minds—Drs. Becker, Farrell and Waller—carefully outline the why and the how of exposure therapy for eating disorders. Essential reading!"
—**Stuart B. Murray**, DClinPsych, PhD, Associate Professor, Department of Psychiatry, University of California, San Francisco

"This text blends state-of-the-art knowledge of the theoretical mechanisms and practical applications of exposure therapy with impressive clinical experience and expertise in the treatment of specific eating disorders. Therapists will find the detailed treatment guidelines and guidance on how to respond to individual patient needs invaluable. It makes a compelling case for the expanded use of exposure therapy and is strongly recommended reading for clinicians treating eating disorders."
—**G. Terence Wilson**, PhD, Oscar K Buros Professor, Graduate School of Applied and Professional Psychology, Rutgers, the State University of New Jersey

ABCT Clinical Practice Series

Series Editor

Susan W. White, Ph.D., ABPP, Professor and Doddridge Saxon Chair in Clinical Psychology, University of Alabama

Associate Editors

Lara J. Farrell, Ph.D., Associate Professor, School of Applied Psychology, Griffith University & Menzies Health Institute of Queensland, Australia

Matthew A. Jarrett, Ph.D., Associate Professor, Department of Psychology, University of Alabama

Jordana Muroff, Ph.D., LICSW, Associate Professor, Clinical Practice, Boston University School of Social Work

Marisol Perez, Ph.D., Associate Professor & Associate Chair, Department of Psychology, Arizona State University

Titles in the Series

Applications of the Unified Protocol for Transdiagnostic Treatment of Emotional Disorders
Edited by David H. Barlow and Todd Farchione

Helping Families of Youth with School Attendance Problems
Christopher A. Kearney

Addressing Parental Accommodation When Treating Anxiety in Children
Eli R. Lebowitz

Exposure Therapy for Child and Adolescent Anxiety and OCD
Stephen P. Whiteside, Thomas H. Ollendick, and Bridget K. Biggs

Exposure Therapy for Eating Disorders

**CAROLYN BLACK BECKER,
NICHOLAS R. FARRELL, AND
GLENN WALLER**

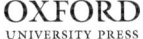

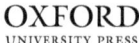

Oxford University Press is a department of the University of Oxford. It furthers
the University's objective of excellence in research, scholarship, and education
by publishing worldwide. Oxford is a registered trade mark of Oxford University
Press in the UK and certain other countries.

Published in the United States of America by Oxford University Press
198 Madison Avenue, New York, NY 10016, United States of America.

© Oxford University Press 2020

All rights reserved. No part of this publication may be reproduced, stored in
a retrieval system, or transmitted, in any form or by any means, without the
prior permission in writing of Oxford University Press, or as expressly permitted
by law, by license, or under terms agreed with the appropriate reproduction
rights organization. Inquiries concerning reproduction outside the scope of the
above should be sent to the Rights Department, Oxford University Press, at the
address above.

You must not circulate this work in any other form
and you must impose this same condition on any acquirer.

Library of Congress Control Number: 2019949811
ISBN 978-0-19-006974-2

In memory of Diana Athey, Jenna Mae Brovold, and Stanley Waller.

CONTENTS

Foreword ix
Preface: Exposure Therapy as a Key Evidence-Based Treatment Strategy for Eating Disorders xi
Acknowledgments xiii
About the Authors xv

PART 1. The Theoretical Basis of Exposure Therapy for Eating Disorders 1

1. Eating Disorders: An Overview 3
2. Overview of Exposure Therapy 11
3. Why Do People Get Better With Exposure Therapy? 19
4. Why Exposure for Eating Disorders? A Rationale for Treatment 33
5. How Well Does Exposure Therapy Work for Eating Disorders? A Summary of the Evidence 45

PART 2. Preparing to Start Exposure Therapy 55

6. Functional Assessment of Eating Disorders and Their Maintenance 57
7. Explaining Exposure Therapy to Your Patients 65
8. Planning Exposure Therapy With Your Patients 77
9. Embarking on Exposure: Important Considerations 89

PART 3. Applying Exposure to Different Eating Disorder Problem Areas 105

10. Exposure to Food and Eating 107
11. Cue Exposure for Binge Eating 121
12. Weighing and Weight Exposure 131
13. Body Image Exposure 141
14. Emotion-Focused and Interpersonal Exposure 155
15. Novel Ways to Use Exposure for Eating Disorders 165

PART 4. Important Considerations in the Delivery of Exposure 173

16. When to Use Cognitive Therapy Techniques to Enhance the Effects of Exposure 175
17. Involving Friends, Family, and Other Loved Ones 185
18. Addressing the Impact of Different Settings and Institutional Resistance 195
19. Dealing With Clinicians' Fears About Using Exposure 205
20. Final Summary: Exposure Therapy in the Treatment of Eating Disorders 213

Appendix—Exposure Therapy: How It Can Help You With Your Eating Disorder 217
References 221
Index 239

FOREWORD

Mental health clinicians desperately want to help their clients and recognize the importance of implementing evidence-based treatments toward achieving this goal. In the past several years, the field of mental healthcare has seen tremendous advances in our understanding of pathology and its underlying mechanisms, as well as proliferation and refinement of scientifically informed treatment approaches. Coinciding with these advances is a heightened focus on accountability in clinical practice. Clinicians are expected to apply evidence-based approaches and to do so effectively, efficiently, and in a patient-centered, individualized way. This is no small order. For a multitude of reasons, including but not limited to client diversity, complex psychopathology (e.g., comorbidity), and barriers to care that are not under the clinician's control (e.g., adverse life circumstances that limit the client's ability to participate), delivery of evidence-based approaches can be challenging.

This series, which represents a collaborative effort between the Association for Behavioral and Cognitive Therapies (ABCT) and the Oxford University Press, is intended to serve as an easy-to-use, highly practical collection of resources for clinicians and trainees. The ABCT Clinical Practice Series is designed to help clinicians effectively master and implement evidence-based treatment approaches. In practical terms, the series represents the "brass tacks" of implementation, including basic how-to guidance and advice on troubleshooting common issues in clinical practice and application. As such, the series is best viewed as a complement to other series on evidence-based protocols such as the Treatments That Work™ series and the Programs That Work™ series. These represent seminal bridges between research and practice and have been instrumental in the dissemination of empirically supported intervention protocols and programs. The ABCT Clinical Practice Series, rather than focusing on specific diagnoses and their treatment, targets the practical application of therapeutic and assessment approaches. In other words, the emphasis is on the how-to aspects of mental health delivery.

It is my hope that clinicians and trainees find these books useful in refining their clinical skills, as enhanced comfort as well as competence in delivery of evidence-based approaches should ultimately lead to improved client outcomes. Given the emphasis on application in this series, there is relatively less emphasis on review of the underlying research base. Readers who wish to delve more deeply into the theoretical or empirical basis supporting specific approaches are encouraged to go to the original-source publications cited in each chapter. When relevant, suggestions for further reading are provided.

EXPOSURE THERAPY FOR EATING DISORDERS

Exposure is a mainstay of effective treatments for eating disorders (ED). Indeed, it is a component of the most well-researched treatment packages. Yet, it is woefully underutilized or implemented in ways that may diminish effectiveness in practice. This book breaks down exposure into its critical elements, while providing an easy-to-use presentation of the theoretical rationale, empirical basis, and clinical rationale for its use. For these reasons, this volume is a highly practical "how to" resource for practicing clinicians and those in training.

On that topic, one of the unique aspects of this volume is the guidance targeted toward clinical supervisors. The authors provide targeted suggestions for helping trainees implement exposure. In summary, this volume will be useful to providers of various disciplines who work with ED patients and to providers at different levels of experience—from trainee to supervisor. It will surely be a useful accompaniment to enrich use of existing ED treatment protocols, as well as a stand-alone resource for clinicians who wish to enrich their understanding and use of exposure.

Drs. Carolyn Black Becker, Nicholas R. Farrell, and Glenn Waller have years of experience—both treating ED patients and conducting research in this area. They have managed to package this immense clinical wisdom into a book that is rich in content yet straightforward, so that clinicians can easily apply the skills conveyed.

Susan W. White, Ph.D., ABPP
Series Editor

PREFACE

Exposure Therapy as a Key Evidence-Based Treatment Strategy for Eating Disorders

Do you have patients who restrict their food intake, binge eat, make themselves vomit, use laxatives or diuretics, engage in unhealthy exercise, hide from emotions, avoid scales and mirrors, repetitively check their body shape, and/or hate talking about eating? If so—this book is for you.

Treating eating disorders (EDs) is a challenge for all clinicians. However, as these disorders have very high personal, health, social, and economic costs (e.g., BEAT, 2015) as well as a high mortality rate (e.g., Arcelus, Mitchell, Wales, & Nielsen, 2011), we collectively need to rise to that challenge. Fortunately, in recent years we have reached a better understanding of what psychological treatments work for patients who have EDs (e.g., National Institute for Health and Care Excellence [NICE], 2017). Importantly, the most effective of these psychotherapies all share a common element; to some degree, each includes *exposure-based therapy*—namely, the directive to guide ED patients in facing their fears. These fears may center around changing eating overall, eating specific foods, gaining weight, learning one's weight, engaging in interpersonal relationships, coping with emotions, seeing one's body, or any of a range of other issues. All of these fears need to be addressed as effectively as possible. The aim of this book is to advance your understanding of exposure therapy so you can more effectively address your patient's fears and anxiety, regardless of which evidence-based treatment you are using.

Exposure therapy (or "exposure with response prevention") was one of the earliest psychotherapies developed. From the start, exposure was based in theory and empirical evidence, emerging from our understanding of both fear acquisition and amelioration. However, thinking about exposure therapy has never stood still, developing well into the 21st century (e.g., Craske, Treanor, Conway, Zbozinek, & Vervliet, 2014). In this book, you will see how both the theory and the existing evidence base supporting exposure have developed over time. This will allow you to be more effective in treating EDs, whether your patient has avoidant/restrictive food intake disorder, anorexia nervosa, bulimia nervosa, binge eating disorder, or an atypical ED presentation (e.g., other specified feeding or eating disorder).

In this book, you will learn

- How an understanding of anxiety underpins developments in our conceptualization and treatment of EDs;
- Why exposure therapy is well-suited to address various features of EDs;
- What the literature tells us about the effectiveness of exposure for different ED-related problem areas;
- The importance of recent developments in exposure therapy for both EDs and anxiety-based disorders;
- How preparing yourself, your trainees, and your patients is an important element of exposure therapy;
- How to use exposure therapy to address specific targets in EDs, such as food avoidance, food triggers, emotional eating, interpersonal fears, body avoidance, and more; and
- How well-meaning families, services, and clinicians can inadvertently get in the way of successful exposure therapy (and how to get past such roadblocks).

The authors are all clinicians and researchers who promote the use of exposure therapy within the treatment of both EDs and anxiety-based disorders. As such, this book includes significant case material, so that you can see exposure therapy in action. In keeping with the nature of this Association for Behavioral and Cognitive Therapies series, we have used the existing evidence base and behavioral theory to develop and support our clinical suggestions. We hope this balance of evidence, theory, and clinical experience will be useful to you every time that you work with an ED patient in helping them to improve and recover.

ACKNOWLEDGMENTS

We are deeply grateful to many people who supported the writing of this book both directly and indirectly. To start, we wish to acknowledge our patients, who have taught us so much about what it is like to both live with and recover from an eating disorder. Their courage and strength is a never-ending source of inspiration. We also would like to thank our mentors and colleagues both for what they have taught us and for putting up with us over the years. Particular mention goes to Brett Deacon, Donn Posner, Kelly Vitousek, and Terry Wilson; we would not be the exposure therapists we are if not for their influence. We thank Francesca Gomez and Bibiana Cutilletta for their assistance in preparing the manuscript for this book. We must note that this book never would have been started were it not for Sarah Harrington at Oxford University Press and Susan White, Series Editor for the Association for Behavioral and Cognitive Therapies. Finally, we want to thank our friends and family, including but not limited to Jennifer Farrell, Michael Farrell, Holly Farrell, and Brent Becker, for all of their support throughout our careers.

ABOUT THE AUTHORS

Carolyn Black Becker is a Professor of Psychology at Trinity University and a licensed clinical psychologist who specializes in the treatment of PTSD, anxiety disorders, and eating disorders. She is board certified in behavioral and cognitive therapy and specializes in the implementation of scientifically supported interventions in clinical and real-world settings. She is a fellow of the Academy for Eating Disorders, the Association for Behavioral and Cognitive Therapies, and the Association for Psychological Science. She currently serves as President of the Society for a Science of Clinical Psychology and is past president of the Academy for Eating Disorders. She has received numerous awards including the Lori Irving Award for Excellence in Eating Disorders Prevention and Awareness granted by the National Eating Disorders Association and the Academy for Eating Disorders Research-Practice Partnership Award.

Nicholas R. Farrell is the clinical director of eating disorders services at Rogers Behavioral Health located in Oconomowoc, Wisconsin. He has expertise in evidence-based psychological treatments, particularly those that emphasize exposure therapy for eating and anxiety disorders. Within this area of expertise, he has published numerous journal articles and book chapters and has given presentations at a variety of international conferences. He has also received grant funding to study stigma reduction efforts among individuals with eating disorders. His research contributions to the field have recently been recognized and awarded by the Academy for Eating Disorders.

Glenn Waller is Professor of Clinical Psychology at the University of Sheffield, United Kingdom. His clinical and academic specialism is evidence-based CBT for eating disorders. He has published over 300 peer-reviewed papers, 20 book chapters, and three books in the field. He regularly presents workshops at national and international meetings. He is past president of the international Academy for Eating Disorders, he is an associate editor of the *International Journal of Eating Disorders*, and he is on the editorial board of *Behaviour Research and Therapy*. He was a member of the NICE Eating Disorders Guideline Development Group, responsible for the 2017 update to the eating disorders guideline.

Exposure Therapy for Eating Disorders

PART 1

The Theoretical Basis of Exposure Therapy for Eating Disorders

1

Eating Disorders

An Overview

Since you have chosen to read this book, you likely have at least a basic understanding of the nature of eating disorders (EDs), as well as some of the different diagnoses in this category. Yet, you may not fully understand the many commonalities shared by different EDs. Perhaps one of the most striking aspects of EDs is how much they remain misunderstood. To illustrate, many members of the general public trivialize EDs as problems of vanity that pale in comparison to the seriousness of other mental health disorders (e.g., depression; Crisp, 2005), even though EDs are extremely severe and debilitating conditions. In addition to being the most lethal of all types of psychiatric disorders (Arcelus, Mitchell, Wales, & Nielsen, 2011), EDs are associated with a wide array of substantial medical complications, such as cardiac abnormalities (e.g., arrhythmias), pancreatitis, and osteoporosis (Westmoreland, Krantz, & Mehler, 2016).

In this chapter, we provide you with an overview of some of the different ED diagnoses and key features of each. However, what is also critical to highlight is the well-established understanding that EDs have more in common with each other than they have features that make them distinct from one another. That is, there are a number of key features that are common across most types of EDs (e.g., Fairburn, Cooper, Shafran, & Wilson, 2008). These transdiagnostic ED features serve as critical targets for exposure-based therapy. We elaborate on these features in the following discussion.

EATING DISORDER DIAGNOSES

Anorexia Nervosa

One of the hallmark features of anorexia nervosa (AN) is severe starvation. This starvation involves limitations to overall volume of daily caloric intake, as well as restriction in the types of food and drink that are consumed. In typical cases, the pattern of restraint in eating leads to either significant weight loss or the absence of appropriate weight gain in the context of normative development.

The pattern of severe starvation in AN is often accompanied by several additional behaviors aimed at lowering weight or curtailing normative weight gain. These include efforts to expel food from the body (e.g., via self-induced vomiting or use of laxatives or diuretic medicines). Many individuals with AN also engage in excessive and unhealthy patterns of exercise designed to burn calories. Later, we will outline how each of these behaviors can be conceptualized as anxiety-reducing behaviors, making them targets for exposure therapy. Finally, while the following are not diagnostic features, it is common for individuals with AN to engage in a wide range of eating-related "safety behaviors" that are designed to decrease anxiety associated with eating (Gianini et al., 2015). Examples include tearing apart food into very small pieces, eating at an abnormally slow pace, making food unpalatable, and excessive wiping of one's mouth and hands with napkins.

Several important features of AN are applicable across the range of ED diagnoses. For instance, while having an intense of fear gaining weight or becoming fat is a diagnostic criterion for AN, it is also common to most other EDs. Likewise, many individuals with AN have extreme body image concerns, which are similarly present in other ED diagnoses.

Bulimia Nervosa

One predominant behavioral manifestation of bulimia nervosa (BN) is recurring episodes of binge eating, in which an individual consumes an abnormally large quantity of food given the circumstances. In many cases, the individual experiencing these episodes perceives a breakdown in her ability to control the content or amount of food and/or the pace at which it is eaten. These binge-eating episodes are often immediately followed by very intense negative emotions, such as guilt over having consumed a large quantity of food and anxiety about consequent changes to weight and body shape.

In an effort to escape from these negative emotions (and prevent the anticipated increases to weight and body shape), individuals with BN engage in maladaptive behavioral responses that are intended to compensate for the calories consumed during the binge. Commonly, these behaviors involve deliberate attempts to expel (i.e., purge) food from the body, such as through self-induced vomiting or abuse of laxatives. There may also be other behaviors that, while not intended to purge food from the body, are nonetheless used in a compensatory manner to "undo" the perceived ill effects of bingeing. Examples of these nonpurging compensatory behaviors include exercising in an obligatory fashion as well as prolonged fasting. Again, such symptoms can be seen as anxiety-reducing behaviors that can be addressed using exposure therapy (see later chapters).

As described in the previous section on AN, individuals with BN also experience several features that are quite pervasive across most ED diagnoses, such as negative body image and extreme anxiety over anticipated weight gain. Again, these symptoms are associated with both *avoidance* (e.g., reducing frequency and caloric content of regular meals, not wearing revealing clothing such as a swimsuit, hiding the body in baggy clothes) and *safety behaviors* (e.g., body checking). Both types of behaviors are aimed at anxiety reduction. This book will not only help you conceptualize and understand these two behavioral patterns, it will help you change them. Another transdiagnostic commonality with AN is semistarvation. Although your BN patients may not be at a low weight, many will experience semistarvation. Semistarvation in both AN and BN is associated with increasingly rigid thinking and less stable emotions. These in turn, drive increased anxiety and further use of avoidance and safety behaviors.

Binge Eating Disorder

Similar to BN, individuals with binge eating disorder (BED) experience repeated episodes of binge eating that are perceived as uncontrollable. There are several key defining characteristics of these binge-eating episodes that are hallmarks of BED. First, in many cases, the individual engages in binge eating despite the absence of feeling hungry at the outset of eating. Relatedly, many individuals with BED report eating food at a very rapid pace during binge episodes, which often results in feeling a great deal of discomfort due to being overly full. Due to the common experience of intense feelings of shame, guilt, and anxiety around these binge-eating episodes, individuals with BED often eat secluded from others. Later, we will outline how binges can serve the function of blocking out emotional states—another form of avoidance where exposure can be a useful tool.

Although there are several aspects of BED that render it distinct from AN and BN (e.g., individuals with BED typically do not engage in compensatory behaviors following binges), it is important to note that BED shares some of the same characteristics that were mentioned in the previous sections on AN and BN. For instance, despite recurrent experiences of overeating, many of your patients with BED will engage in periodic dieting and experience consistent fluctuations in their weight. The tendency to overemphasize body size in influencing one's self-concept that is present in AN and BN is also very common among individuals diagnosed with BED (Grilo et al., 2009). Finally, BED often involves a comparable degree of preoccupation and disturbance with body image to that observed in AN and BN (Ahrberg, Trojca, Nasrawi, & Vocks, 2011).

Avoidant/Restrictive Food Intake Disorder

A new diagnosis to *Diagnostic and Statistical Manual of Mental Disorders–Fifth Edition* (DSM-5; American Psychiatric Association, 2013), avoidant/restrictive food intake disorder (ARFID) is marked by significant limitations to one's overall dietary intake. On the surface, the restrictive eating habits in ARFID appear to closely resemble the severe starvation that is characteristic of AN. However, whereas individuals with AN practice restraint in their eating due to concerns surrounding their physique, the eating-related avoidance seen in ARFID is typically done out of fear of experiencing significant negative consequences (e.g., choking, uncontrollable vomiting) or anxiety in response to aversive sensory/physical experiences related to eating. Anxiety is a strong feature of ARFID, making it amenable to exposure-based approaches (e.g., Nicholls, Christie, Randall, & Lask, 2001).

One notable absence from typical ARFID features is the body image-related disturbances that are often quite prominent in AN, BN, and BED. Unlike the previously described EDs, individuals with ARFID do not possess intense fears of weight gain or becoming fat. On the contrary, you will find that many of your patients with ARFID will be quite distressed at their perceived inability to maintain a biologically appropriate weight and would happily gain weight if given the opportunity to do so. Other aspects of ARFID that set it apart somewhat from other EDs involve the demographic makeup of those diagnosed with ARFID. Unlike most other EDs, there appear to be just as many males diagnosed with ARFID as females (Nicely, Lane-Loney, Masciulli, Hollenbeak, & Ornstein, 2014). Additionally, ARFID is a problem that tends to affect children and adolescents more frequently than it does adults.

Other Specified/Unspecified Eating Disorders

In past editions of the *Diagnostic and Statistical Manual of Mental Disorders,* individuals who experienced ED symptoms that did not "fit" neatly into any of the other ED diagnostic categories were given a diagnosis of eating disorder not otherwise specified (EDNOS). Given the highly varied presentation of ED symptoms from one patient to the next, the EDNOS diagnosis was used frequently (e.g., Fairburn & Harrison, 2003). In the DSM-5 (American Psychiatric Association, 2013), symptom presentations that involve clinically significant ED features without completely fulfilling the diagnostic criteria of other ED diagnoses are assigned a diagnosis of either other specified feeding or eating disorder(OSFED) or unspecified feeding or eating disorder. Like EDNOS, these two categories are together something of a catch-all diagnostic classification. This designation, right or wrong, should not diminish the substantial impact these conditions can have. For instance, individuals with atypical AN meet all criteria for AN with the exception that, despite significant weight loss, actual weight remains above or at normal levels. Purging disorder also may involve similar levels of purging to BN, but there is an absence of binge eating. Put simply, the nonspecific ED diagnoses are not any less distressing than the specific ones, and anxiety and avoidant/safety behaviors are just as likely to need to be addressed in such cases.

A QUICK WORD ON OTHER EATING DISORDERS

There are other ED diagnoses that we have chosen not to review in this chapter, such as rumination disorder and pica. Our intention is not to diminish the importance of these problems, but they are (a) less common disorders and (b) relatively unlikely to present at ED-oriented treatment settings. Furthermore, these disorders are less clearly rooted in anxiety and share few of the transdiagnostic ED features that are the central targets of exposure-based interventions.

KEY TRANSDIAGNOSTIC FEATURES OF EATING DISORDERS

Although knowledge of the different ED diagnoses is an important foundation, you will find that having an understanding of the key features that span ED diagnoses is essential to effectively using exposure for EDs (e.g., the fact that an individual's diagnosis changes from AN to BN does not make exposure any less relevant). More specifically, as previously alluded to, despite the significant heterogeneity of ED symptom presentations, you will discover that transdiagnostic features (e.g., food avoidance, body image disturbance) are consistent common threads running through your patients' EDs. It is worth noting that there is a well-established precedent for conceptualizing and treating EDs from a transdiagnostic perspective, with particular emphasis on key features like food avoidance and body image (e.g., Wade, Bergin, Martin, Gillespie, & Fairburn, 2006).

In the following sections, we provide some additional discussion covering three of the most critical transdiagnostic ED features to which many exposure techniques apply. We will expand on these overviews in later chapters that cover application of exposure to these transdiagnostic problem areas. First, consider the following case example that encompasses each of these three features.

> Monica, a 22-year-old college student, sought treatment for an ED. She described herself as a pudgy kid who was often teased by her peers about her weight. When she began high school, her older sister helped her begin dieting while also introducing her to regular exercise. She lost 25 pounds over the next several months and noticed that her peers stopped teasing her.
>
> Monica continued dieting but noticed that she stopped losing weight. She then began to significantly restrict her daily food intake, which consisted of eating meager portions at meals while also cutting out any snacking. She and her friends also began to do monthly "cleanses," during which they would fast for one or two days. Monica began to weigh herself each morning and developed a rule that she would skip breakfast if her weight had increased at all from the previous day.
>
> Entering college, Monica became increasingly preoccupied with her weight and body shape. She ate only when she could no longer ignore her hunger, and she joined a fitness group on campus that met daily to engage

in vigorous cardiovascular exercise. She also began to engage in frequent body-checking behaviors. While under stress studying for her end-of-year exams, Monica had a binge-eating episode in which she rapidly ate an entire package of chocolate cookies while also occasionally spooning peanut butter into her mouth. Feeling horrified about what she had done, she immediately stopped studying and went to the gym to exercise until she felt she had "undone" those calories.

As college went on, Monica followed a similar pattern of restricting her daily food intake while also exercising vigorously. She continued to experience periodic binge-eating episodes (on average once every 3–4 weeks), which continued to provoke intense feelings of anxiety and shame. Although Monica's weight remained slightly lower than her biologically appropriate range, her primary care physician did not express any concern during her routine appointments because she had not lost her menstrual cycle or encountered any other significant medical red flags.

Eating-Related Fear and Avoidance

In the previous example, Monica shows fairly typical eating-related fear and the subsequent avoidance behaviors that are common across ED diagnoses. Many individuals with EDs fear that eating too much food and/or certain types of forbidden foods will cause exorbitant, uncontrollable weight gain, a belief that is central to many forms of ED pathology (Waller & Mountford, 2015). Although weight gain (or, at times, weight maintenance in patients unable to lose weight) is likely the most common feared outcome that patients with EDs endorse, remember that eating-related fears in EDs extend beyond the realm of weight gain. To illustrate, a patient with ARFID may fear eating food in normal-sized bites in anticipation of choking. Other ARFID fears include fear that eating certain types of food will lead to a medical catastrophe, such as experiencing anaphylactic shock or congestive heart failure. The specific nature of patients' eating-related fears often predicts the types of avoidant and safety behaviors they use to try to prevent feared outcomes (Levinson et al., 2018). For instance, patients fearful of weight gain may restrict their caloric intake and engage in compulsory exercise between meals. In contrast, patients who fear choking may consume food at an exceeding slow pace, take abnormally small bites of food, and chew excessively before swallowing.

Body Image Disturbance

A large body of literature attests to the central role of body image disturbance in the development and maintenance of ED pathology (e.g., Rohde, Stice, & Marti,

2015), as well as in the occurrence of relapse following ostensibly successful treatment (Keel, Dorer, Franko, Jackson, & Herzog, 2005). This is certainly illustrated in the case of Monica, who exhibits clear problems with accepting and tolerating disliked aspects of her physique. As with many ED patients, Monica's anxiety about her body manifests in several body-focused behaviors aimed at reducing anxiety. Notably, body checking, which is a safety behavior, and body image avoidance (e.g., wearing exceedingly baggy clothing to hide the body) are common transdiagnostic ED behaviors that have shown to play a central role in the expression and maintenance of EDs (e.g., Trottier, MacDonald, McFarlane, Carter, & Olmsted, 2015).

Binge Eating

As reviewed earlier in the chapter, binge eating is a feature that is present across ED diagnoses but is most commonly observed in BN and BED. Individuals with these diagnoses often experience a similar degree of body image disturbance and consequent dieting behaviors to that experienced by individuals with AN. It follows that individuals' dieting over time directly contributes to uncontrollable episodes of binge eating. Indeed, many individuals diagnosed with BED report extensive histories of varied dieting "successes," only to have these periods followed by recurrent binge eating and often substantial weight gain. In addition to continual dieting, other contributors to binge eating include stimuli that have become conditioned cues for bingeing by virtue of their being repeatedly paired with binge episodes (see Chapter 11 for in-depth discussion). That is, various physical and emotional antecedents to binge eating can develop the power to elicit a conditioned response of strong binge-eating cravings (Jansen & van den Hout, 1991). Examples of common cues that elicit binge-eating cravings for ED patients include various forms of interacting with food, such as seeing, smelling, and tasting food. Negative emotional experiences that frequently precede binge episodes can also become a powerful stimulus that elicits binge cravings (Bongers & Jansen, 2017).

SUMMARY

EDs are serious mental health disorders that are associated with significant morbidity and mortality. When treating EDs, you need a good understanding of both the differences associated with specific ED diagnoses and the transdiagnostic features that commonly present across diagnoses. Many, if not all, of the common features can be targeted using exposure therapy as will be discussed in subsequent chapters.

2

Overview of Exposure Therapy

WHAT IS EXPOSURE THERAPY?

On the surface, exposure therapy is a very straightforward technique. First, you identify things or situations that your patient fears. Most often your patient will have a history of avoiding the stimuli you identify or only tolerating them in the context of safety cues (e.g., going to a feared location with a safe person). Next, you and your patient collaboratively choose a specific starting stimulus. Finally, you purposefully expose your patient to the feared stimulus, often repeatedly and/or for a prolonged period of time. Exposure is quite intuitive for most people. Indeed, we see a basic understanding of exposure in common adages, including advice to "face your fears" and the saying "You need to get back on the horse if you fall off."

Research supports this common sense understanding of the utility of exposure, particularly for the treatment of anxiety-based disorders. For instance, exposure serves as the backbone for cognitive-behavioral therapy (CBT) for panic disorder (Craske & Barlow, 2007); CBT for panic disorder is widely recognized as a first-line treatment (McHugh, Smits, & Otto, 2009). Exposure also underpins efficacious variants of CBT for social anxiety disorder, specific phobia, obsessive-compulsive disorder (OCD) and posttraumatic stress disorder (PTSD; American Psychological Association, 2017; Choy, Fyer, & Lipsitz, 2007; Olatunji, Cisler, Deacon, 2010; Öst, Havnen, Hansen, & Kvale, 2015; Ponniah & Hollon, 2008). In this book, we will show you that exposure is just as central to the understanding and treatment of eating disorders (EDs). However, because exposure has been most widely studied and used in the treatment of anxiety-based disorders, it is useful for us to consider the use of exposure for patients with pathological anxiety before expanding our discussion to EDs in subsequent chapters. You will be a better ED exposure clinician if you have a basic understanding of the myriad of ways in which exposure is used to address anxiety-based disorders.

As will be discussed further in Chapter 4, a key aim of exposure therapy is for your patient to learn that (a) he can tolerate anxiety to a greater degree than anticipated and (b) his expectation that a situation or stimulus is truly dangerous is incorrect (Craske et al., 2008). The latter is often described as *safety learning*. The case of Kara demonstrates just a few of the ways in which exposure can be used to teach these lessons for anxiety associated with different disorders.

> Kara, a 28-year old mother of two boys, met criteria for PTSD secondary to a sexual assault that occurred when she served in the military. She also met criteria for OCD and panic disorder. Kara's OCD fears stemmed from obsessions regarding contamination and included an obsession that she would be "contaminated" by and die from botulism poisoning. Kara's diet largely consisted of toasted white bread and tomato soup, the latter of which had to be brought to a rolling boil for a minimum of 30 minutes to "kill the botulism." Kara reported knowing her obsession about botulism poisoning did not, in her words, "make sense" because she was willing to feed her sons and husband other foods even though she loved them and would never do anything to risk their health. Kara experienced both unexpected panic attacks and attacks triggered by other situations that made her anxious. For instance, on the rare occasions when she tried to eat a feared food, Kara often experienced a panic attack, which she then interpreted as confirmation that the food had contaminated or "sickened" her.
>
> Kara's treatment, which was highly successful, involved exposure to a wide variety of stimuli. For example, to address her obsessions about contamination, Kara's clinician exposed her to touching feared objects, sitting on "contaminated" surfaces, and eating feared foods. Kara agreed to not engage in washing or decontamination rituals before, during, or after exposure so she could both learn to tolerate her anxiety and discover whether feared outcomes (e.g., dying of botulism or contracting rabies) actually occurred. Kara's primary care physician wanted her to take a multivitamin because her diet was so nutrient poor, but Kara feared the vitamin could be a source of salmonella. So, Kara also completed vitamin exposure. To address her panic attacks, Kara participated in exposure to feared physiological sensations (e.g., shortness of breath, dizziness). To create the sensations, Kara's clinician instructed her to hyperventilate, breathe through a straw, and spin in a chair. Later, Kara watched scary movies in a hot room while bundled up in a coat after drinking two cups of coffee. Kara also engaged in driving exposure to learn that she could successfully drive a car, even while having a panic attack. Through this, Kara again learned she was better able to tolerate anxiety than anticipated; she also learned that symptoms of a panic attack did not mean she was about to pass out or die.
>
> PTSD treatment often includes both exposure to memories of the traumatic experience and exposure to stimuli that are associated with the traumatic event(s) in some way. Exposure to memories is sometimes misinterpreted as making patients "relive" their traumatic experience. Instead, the aim is for patients to discover that although the original event was dangerous, the memory of the event is not dangerous. Kara completed exposure to her

> memory of being raped by a fellow military officer. She also completed exposure to the soap her perpetrator made her use to clean up after the rape, as well as other trauma-related stimuli that triggered her fear.

TYPES OF EXPOSURE

As highlighted by Kara's case, there are many different types of exposure that are used to treat a range of disorders. In the following discussion, we provide a brief overview of the most common forms of exposure.

In Vivo Exposure

In vivo (i.e., in reality) exposure is the most common form of exposure and involves exposing your patient to the actual stimuli or situation that evokes fear. If your patient fears spiders, snakes, or heights and you use actual spiders, snakes, or elevated situations during exposure, you are conducting in vivo exposure. In vivo exposure is commonly used in the treatment of specific phobias. As demonstrated in the case of Kara, it also is a critical component in the treatment of panic disorder (e.g., driving exposure or watching scary movies), OCD (e.g., eating feared foods and touching contaminated surfaces), and even PTSD (e.g., exposure to soap). Further, in vivo exposure is commonly used in treatment of social anxiety. Traditionally, exposure for social anxiety has been designed to teach patients that feared negative social outcomes are unlikely to happen (e.g., people are unlikely to laugh at them) and that they will be able to handle social situations even when anxious. More recently, however, in vivo exposure for social anxiety has extended to social mishap exposure, in which patients are deliberately exposed to their feared negative social outcomes. This is done by having patients behave in ways that make them appear strange, incompetent, rude, etc. (Fang, Sawyer, Asnaani & Hofmann, 2013). There is some evidence that social mishap exposure is the most potent form of in vivo exposure for reducing social anxiety (Nelson, Deacon, Lickel, & Sy, 2010).

Imaginal Exposure

Although you will be able to address many of your patients' fears with in vivo exposure, some situations are not amenable to in vivo work. As previously noted we do not want to re-expose PTSD patients to actually being raped or assaulted. We also do not want to burn down their homes, crash their cars, or flood their towns. Rather, we want PTSD patients to realize that their *memories* are not dangerous, even though the original events were dangerous. To do this, we use imaginal exposure. In imaginal exposure for PTSD, patients optimally close their eyes and describe their memory of their traumatic event in detail repeatedly (see Foa, Hembree, & Rothbaum, 2007). Patients are instructed to close their eyes so they can become more immersed in their memory. In doing so they (a) learn they can tolerate the anxiety associated with remembering; (b) learn that the memory cannot hurt them, even though it is deeply unpleasant; and (c) create a coherent narrative of their traumatic memory. Creating such a narrative helps patients "process" their traumatic experiences, which are often chaotic and overwhelming (see Zayfert & Becker, in press, for additional detail). For your patients who are deeply ashamed or who feel guilty about what they did or did not do during a traumatic event, they also learn that you, their clinician, still care about them and are not revolted, even though you know their "secret." In other words, for these patients, part of imaginal exposure involves in vivo exposure to the fear of sharing what happened with someone.

Imaginal exposure is also used in the treatment of OCD when it is not possible to otherwise expose your patient to the content of an obsession. The case of Darryl provides an example of the use of imaginal exposure.

> Darryl, a 40-year old married man, met criteria for OCD. Darryl's obsession centered around images of stabbing his wife, whom he deeply loved. Although Darryl made some progress with in vivo exposure to knives, which he had avoided since developing this particular obsession, he still engaged in mental rituals (i.e., covert compulsions) to push the image of stabbing his wife from his mind whenever it occurred. More specifically, Darryl would say three Hail Mary prayers and imagine parts of his wedding day until he "felt right."
>
> Darryl made substantially more progress after embarking on imaginal exposure. For Darryl, imaginal exposure involved deliberately imagining stabbing his wife, while resisting the urge to engage in his neutralizing rituals (i.e., response prevention of his compulsions). For patients who have harming obsessions, it can be helpful to start with placing the clinician in the position of being the one imaginably harmed. For instance, Darryl was initially incapable of conducting imaginal exposure to the image of stabbing his wife. So the clinician inquired if Darryl would find it anxiety-provoking to imagine stabbing the clinician and whether he would want to neutralize such an image. Imaginal exposure to stabbing his clinician was less anxiety-provoking but still challenging for Darryl, and it served as a successful stepping stone to imaginal exposure to stabbing his wife.

Although exposure often plays a smaller role in treatment of generalized anxiety disorder (GAD), imaginal exposure is also used with GAD patients (Hoyer & Beesdo-Baum, 2012). Worrying in GAD is conceptualized as a cognitive avoidance behavior that prevents critical processing of thoughts and images behind the worry (Borkovec, Alcaine, & Behar, 2004). For instance, consider the case of Kimiko.

> Kimiko worried extensively about her university course work. Kimiko's clinician encouraged Kimiko to share her deepest fear related to doing poorly in school. Ultimately Kimiko described a scenario in which she first failed an exam, which then led to failing a class, which ultimately led to further failing, dropping out of university, being disowned by her parents, and ending up homeless. Kimiko then created a worry scenario, with the help of her clinician, in which this worst fear happened. Exposure involved vividly imagining the scenario actually happening, while describing the scenario in detail out loud. Kimiko's clinician audio recorded this session, and Kimiko subsequently used the audio recording to facilitate home practice of imaginal exposure.

Interoceptive Exposure

As demonstrated with Kara, the aim of interoceptive exposure is to replicate and systematically expose patients to feared physiological sensations associated with panic or anxiety. Standard brief exercises used to evoke such sensations include, but are not limited to, running in place (or doing step ups or jumping jacks), muscle tension, holding one's breath, head shaking, breathing through a thin straw, spinning, using a tongue depressor, and hyperventilating (Craske & Barlow, 2007). Although interoceptive exposure is most commonly used in the treatment of panic disorder, it may also be used in the treatment of other anxiety problems that are accompanied by feared physical sensations. Indeed, the trait of anxiety sensitivity (i.e., a fear of anxiety-related sensations; Reiss, 1991), which is theoretically targeted by interoceptive exposure, has been proposed as a transdiagnostic risk factor for the development of anxiety-based disorders (Boswell et al., 2013).

For instance, social phobia is often accompanied by outwardly observable anxiety symptoms that are perceived by patients as having negative social consequences (e.g., blushing, sweating, trembling). Dixon, Kemp, Farrell, Blakey, and Deacon (2015) identified additional exercises beyond the standard ones for panic disorder that can be useful in evoking these physical symptoms commonly associated with social anxiety. Sample exercises include applying heat to one's face, eating hot sauce, doing push-ups, and consuming a hot drink. Interoceptive exposure also may be useful in the treatment of PTSD because physiological sensations frequently accompany traumatic experiences (Wald & Taylor, 2007; 2008). Some sensations occur secondary to fear; others, as in the case of Damian, result directly from the trauma, such as sensations associated with being choked, smothered, or held down.

> Damian had been forcibly held on the ground by police when he was mistakenly identified as a suspect in a crime. During this time, Damian feared that the police might shoot him. He also experienced difficulty breathing because one officer sat on him, while another handcuffed him. Damian experienced intense anxiety any time he felt his breathing might be constricted and was so frightened of this situation that he would not let his girlfriend hug him. Damian's clinician used traditional interoceptive breathing exercises to replicate the sense of being smothered (e.g., straw breathing). She also had Damian lie under multiple heavy blankets to replicate the sensation of a weight impairing his breathing. Damian's case demonstrates the need to sometimes be creative in finding ways to produce feared physiological sensations.

Virtual Reality Exposure

Virtual reality exposure (i.e., exposure using computer generated simulation of a virtual environment) is increasingly an affordable option for clinicians, thanks to the development of low-cost devices that can produce immersive experiences (Bun, Gorski, Grajewski, Wichniarek, & Zawadzki, 2017). Most commonly, virtual reality exposure has been tested with specific phobias, social anxiety disorder, and PTSD (Parsons & Rizzo, 2008). Virtual reality exposure is a potential option when in vivo exposure is viewed as ideal but is not feasible or would be difficult to implement. For instance, particularly post the September 11th attacks, it is very difficult, if not impossible, for clinicians to access behind security portions of airports to conduct exposure with patients who have a fear of flying that has generalized to airports. Clearly, most clinicians also do not have access to actual airplanes so that patients can complete exposure to actually flying. Therefore, it is not surprising that flying phobia is one of the most commonly studied problems in virtual reality exposure. Virtual reality is also an option for your patients who fear heights or driving and as an alternative to keeping actual spiders or snakes in your office. Virtual reality exposure research is in its infancy compared to research into in vivo, imaginal, and interoceptive exposure. It is beyond the scope of this chapter to review this growing literature in detail. Nonetheless, it is important to consider the level of empirical support before embarking on this approach (see Botella, Serrano, Baños, & Garcia-Palacios, 2015; Gonçalves, Pedrozo, Coutinho, Figueira & Ventura, 2012; Meyerbröker, & Emmelkamp, 2010, for sample reviews).

SUMMARY

Exposure is an extremely powerful technique for reducing pathological anxiety. As demonstrated in this chapter, this very common-sense strategy can be adapted to address a wide range of anxiety-based disorders. Although the efficacy of exposure has been long recognized, researchers and clinicians continue to find new ways to adapt exposure to more effectively address anxiety and barriers to treatment.

Why Do People Get Better With Exposure Therapy?

To optimally help your patients using exposure therapy, you need a clear understanding of the possible mechanisms underpinning exposure. Unfortunately, no one knows for sure exactly how or why exposure works (Hofmann, 2008). In addition (and adding complexity), exposure likely works for slightly different reasons for different patients. As noted by Craske, Treanor, Conway, Zbozinek, and Vervliet (2014), exposure works when your patient learns what your patient needs to learn. To this point, different patients need to learn different things. In this chapter, we use the case of Miquel to explore both historical and more contemporary perspectives as to how exposure works. Although no one can say definitively that any one model is completely correct, the models we emphasize are backed by empirical evidence and can help you make clinical decisions so that you optimize the chance for your patients to learn what they need to learn.

> Miquel, a 25-year-old married father of two children, formerly worked retail in a department store and supplemented his family's income by driving for a ride sharing service. Approximately 2 years ago, his car was hit by a bus when he was returning home from working his ride-sharing job. Miquel was severely injured and spent 2 months in hospital, followed by 3 months in a rehabilitation facility. Since discharge, Miquel has been unable to return to either of his jobs because of a profound fear of driving or riding in a car. Miquel even finds it difficult to sit in his new car when the car is turned off in the garage.
>
> Since the crash, Miquel has gained a significant amount of weight secondary to both binge eating and decreased exercise. Miquel reported that he was always the "chunkiest" in his family and worked hard to keep his weight "normal" via a very strict diet and running program. However, severe residual pain in both of his legs and back forced him to give up running, and he began gaining weight. Depressed about both his inability to support his family ("I was always very good at taking care of my family") and changes

> in his body, Miquel began binge eating. He notes that this is his only way to "block everything out," at least in the short term. Miquel's family has a history of drug and alcohol use problems, and he reports being determined not to get "hooked" on either. Miquel's wife is frustrated by his inability to travel by car and stressed about finances, which has led to arguments.

UNLEARNING, HABITUATION, SYSTEMATIC DESENSITIZATION, AND INHIBITORY LEARNING

To understand what Miquel needs to learn as a result of exposure, we first need to explore what Miquel learned as a result of his car crash. Traumatic events like car crashes are typically easier examples to use when initially considering different models about what learning needs to happen during exposure. Once you have an understanding of the different models, you will be able to easily apply them to EDs.

Prior to the car crash, Miquel viewed cars as relatively safe. During the car crash, Miquel learned that the broad concept of "cars" (particularly when impacted by a large bus!) can be associated with profound danger; indeed, he nearly died. After the car crash, Miquel rigidly holds onto to his new understanding of cars as very dangerous, even when the car is safe in his garage. Note that although Miquel learned to view cars as very dangerous because of an actual car crash, humans easily learn fear and anxiety via a variety of mechanisms—not just direct experience (Rachman, 1977). For instance, we can learn fear by observing other people's fear of a situation. We can also learn via "information transmission" (e.g., reading an article about a plane crash). This makes sense. You don't want to have to actually experience being burned by fire to figure out that fire is dangerous. Similarly, your low-weight patients don't have to gain socially unacceptable amounts of weight to feel anxious about not conforming to societal weight standards. Importantly, no matter how your patients learn to maladaptively fear something, exposure can help them address that fear.

Unlearning Model

Original models of exposure, which were based on classical conditioning, posited that fears are "extinguished" or "unlearned" during exposure, when the feared (but reasonably safe) stimulus is repeatedly paired with the absence of actual danger. According to this model, if Miquel engages in car exposure by repeatedly sitting in, riding in, and driving cars, he will unlearn his fear of cars and driving. We now know this is incorrect. We never completely unlearn fear or anxiety, and Miquel will never fully unlearn the association of cars with pain, fear, and actual danger. We know this because successfully treated (or extinguished) fears often

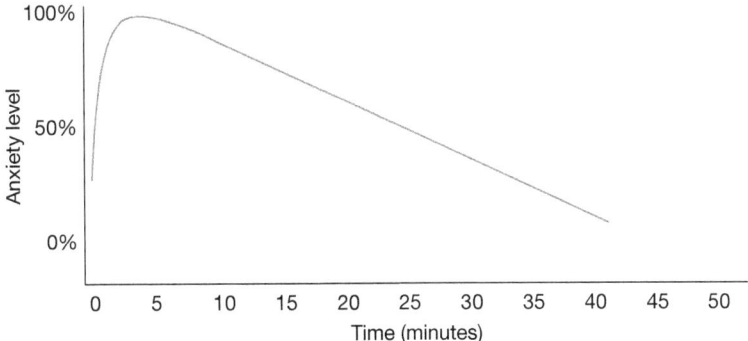

Figure 3.1. Within-session habituation, showing anxiety rising at the beginning of exposure, then falling over time.

spontaneously return (Vervliet, Craske, & Hermans, 2013). Clearly, the learning never went away.

Emotional Processing Theory (i.e., the Habituation Model)

Another perspective regarding the learning that takes place during exposure is emotional processing theory, or what is often referred to as the habituation model (Foa & Kozak, 1986; Foa & McNally, 1996). According to this perspective, if Miquel engages in car exposure for a sufficient amount of time, he will learn that his anxiety will naturally subside (as long as he gives it enough time). This natural reduction of anxiety is referred to as habituation. You can think of this as a sort of "burnout" model. Key learning, according to this model, is that anxiety does not go on forever if the situation is actually safe. You just have to wait it out.

Habituation can occur in two different ways. Within-session habituation refers to the anxiety reduction that frequently occurs during a single session of exposure (see Figure 3.1). Between-session habituation occurs across trials (see Figure 3.2).

If Miquel's clinician was using the habituation model for in vivo car exposure, she would construct a "hierarchy" of feared car- and crash-related experiences, ordered from weaker to stronger fears. The hierarchy serves as a map of the wide variety of situations that trigger Miquel's fear. In addition to car-related situations, Miquel avoids listening to the type of music that was playing when his car was hit. He also covers his ears whenever an ambulance drives by with sirens on. These situations would be included in Miquel's hierarchy.

> **Clinician:** So as we discussed, we need to get a sense of the degree to which different types of car-related experiences cause you anxiety. You mentioned that even looking at cars in magazines makes you anxious, but that photos are also not as bad as other car situations. So let's start there. On a scale of zero to 100—how anxious do car photos make you?

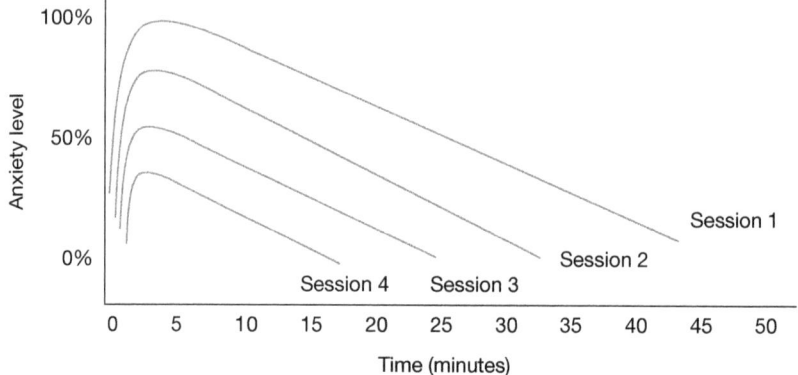

Figure 3.2. Between-session habituation, showing differences in initial and peak levels of anxiety and rates of decline, over several exposure sessions.

Miquel: Not too terrible. Say a 25.

Miquel's clinician has him rate his anxiety using a zero-to-100 rating scale of subjective units of distress (SUDs). This allows Miquel and his clinician to assess the relative intensity of his predicted anxiety in different situations and during the course of exposure. SUDs ratings also can be used for other emotions and are used with other CBT techniques (e.g., cognitive restructuring) to assess the intensity of a particular emotion. You do not have to use a zero-to-100 scale, but it intuitively works for many patients.

Clinician: Great. So let's think about the other end of the scale. What would be the most anxiety-provoking?
Miquel: That is easy. Driving by myself, on the same highway where that bus hit me. That is like 100 plus. Even worse with music on. . . .
Clinician: Okay. Now let's fill in the middle rungs so we can figure out where to start.

After constructing the hierarchy, the clinician and Miquel collaboratively decide what situation or stimuli to use to start in vivo exposure. All forms of exposure can be conducted in either a graduated or intensive fashion. In graduated exposure, the patient moves up the rungs of the hierarchy ladder, starting with easier exposure situations and then moving on to more difficult exposure situations. The presumption is that successful completion of lower exposure tasks makes completing more difficult tasks easier.

Alternatively, Miquel and his clinician could jump to the top of his hierarchy. This is referred to as intensive exposure or flooding. The advantage of this approach is that it can be a much faster way to engage in exposure. If your patient can tolerate this approach, he could improve faster. The disadvantage is that many patients are simply unwilling to approach their most highly feared situations until they have success with exposure (and many clinicians are just as reluctant; see Chapter 19). Further, if the anxiety is too intense and your patient flees from exposure, she will not have a successful learning experience. Getting her to re-engage with exposure after fleeing may prove tricky if not impossible. However, sometimes you have no choice but to go the intensive route because *everything* is highly anxiety-provoking.

If you take the graduated approach, the typical recommended starting point is somewhere around 50 SUDs—high enough on the hierarchy to lead to significant anxiety but low enough to seem doable. Many clinicians collude with their patients' avoidant tendencies by agreeing to start very low on the hierarchy. This allows clinicians to avoid the anxiety that *they* (i.e., clinicians) experience when their patients become distressed. You should attend to indicators that you might be unintentionally colluding. Such collusion is problematic for three reasons:

> **Reasons why you should not collude with your patients in avoiding their (and your) anxiety:**
>
> - A key task of exposure according to the habituation model is for your patients to experience the natural cessation of anxiety that occurs when they stay in even a very anxiety-provoking situation. Your patients cannot have this learning experience if they do not actually experience significant anxiety.
> - It is unethical to let your own anxiety stop you from offering a highly effective form of treatment to your patient.
> - This "low and slow" approach to exposure is inefficient, prolonging your patient's suffering and increasing the amount therapy costs.

One way to explain the inefficiency issue to your patients is using a diving board analogy (Zayfert & Becker, in press).

> **Clinician:** So imagine that you wanted to be able to dive off this high diving board, but you were really scared to dive at all.
> **Miquel:** Okay.
> **Clinician:** Now you could start by standing on the edge of the pool, crouching down into a tight tuck, and then rolling into the pool, which you don't find terribly anxiety-provoking. You could do that repeatedly until you felt really comfortable. Then you could loosen that tuck and repeat until you felt really comfortable. Then you could practice diving from the edge until you felt really comfortable. Then you could baby step your way to higher and higher platforms making sure you are really comfortable before proceeding to the next step. What do you think of this plan?
> **Miquel:** Seems like it would take a really long time.

Clinician: Agreed. What do you think would be a better plan?
Miquel: Well I should probably start with something that is hard, not too easy, but that I can do.

Miquel and his clinician chose sitting in an unmoving, turned-off car to start. They began using Miquel's wife's car parked in the clinic parking lot. Having his clinician in the car during the first session of exposure reduced Miquel's anxiety to a tolerable but still high level. It also made it possible for Miquel's clinician to observe Miquel during the exposure and to provide suggestions for engaging with the exposure. According to the habituation model, Miquel should not try to distract himself from his anxiety.

Clinician: So as we discussed before, we are going to sit in the car for an extended period of time. At least 60 minutes or until your anxiety drops by at least 50%—remember that graph I drew you where the anxiety went up fast and then came back down slowly?
Miquel: Yes, I remember.
Clinician: Great. Also remember that you need to feel the anxiety for it to drop naturally on its own. So if you ask me for reassurance that being in the car is safe, I am going to tell you to just experience your anxiety. Remember that it is really important to stick with your anxiety and not distract yourself or try to force it down.
Miquel: Okay. And I have to do this again, right? You said once is not enough.
Clinician: That is correct. As we discussed, we call the drop in anxiety that occurs in a single session within-session habituation. But every time you do this, it will get easier. We call that between-session habituation. Research suggests that between-session habituation is more important than within-session habituation. So if your anxiety does not come down a lot in this first session, don't worry about that. That is okay. Most people experience within-session habituation, but between-session habituation is more important.
Miquel: Okay. How do we start?
Clinician: Now we are going to get in the car. You agreed to sit behind the steering wheel, and I will sit next to you.
Both Miquel and Clinician get in car.
Clinician: So on a scale of zero to 100, where is your anxiety right now?
Miquel: Sixty-five. I don't like this.
Clinician: That is understandable. We are just going to sit here so you can feel your anxiety. Remember, anxiety is just a feeling; it can't actually hurt you.

As Miquel's clinician notes in the previous dialogue, between-session habituation (i.e., reduction in anxiety across trials) appears to be more important for long-term anxiety reduction than within-session habituation (Rauch & Foa, 2006). However, because most patients experience within-session habituation, when using this model clinicians typically set the expectation that anxiety is very likely to subside within a single session of exposure. Yet, because not all patients experience within-session habituation—even those who respond to exposure using this model—it is important to let your patient know it is okay if he does not experience within-session habituation.

NOTE: SYSTEMATIC DESENSITIZATION IS NOT EXPOSURE

We have frequently heard ED clinicians refer to "desensitization" in the treatment of EDs. Thus, we want to clarify that systematic desensitization is not exposure. Systematic desensitization refers to an early behavioral treatment for anxiety disorders that trained patients in relaxation and then paired the relaxed state with the feared situation or stimuli (Davison, 1968). The rationale behind systematic desensitization was that the relaxed state was incompatible with feeling anxious, and the goal was to condition the relaxed state to the feared stimuli. Systematic desensitization was largely abandoned because exposure is significantly more effective and efficient in the treatment of anxiety. The lesson that systematic desensitization teaches us is that making exposure to anxiety-provoking stimuli less anxiety-inducing makes that exposure less effective. That becomes very relevant when understanding the next model (inhibitory learning) and its implications for conducting exposure work.

INHIBITORY LEARNING MODEL

Many patients have benefited from exposure therapy delivered according to the habituation model, and many features of exposure per the habituation model still make good sense (e.g., using a hierarchy to map out and organize your patients' many fears, encouraging patients to experience their anxiety to the fullest, and *not* going "low and slow"). Nonetheless, Craske et al. (2014) have proposed that exposure effects could be further enhanced if exposure is delivered according to the inhibitory learning model as opposed to the habituation model. They argue that research does not support various aspects of the habituation model including, as previously noted, the importance of within-session habituation (see Craske et al., 2008, 2014, for more detailed discussion). We should note that the jury is still out regarding the utility of both within-session and between-session exposure. Although it is beyond the scope of this book to discuss this in detail, recent research by Benito et al. (2018) suggests that the failure of within-session habituation to predict outcome may be an artifact of measurement problems, as well as the natural tendency of both clinicians and patients to "up the ante" and make exposure harder as patients feel more comfortable with the task. They are not alone in raising concerns about the challenge of accurately measuring all forms of habituation (e.g., Sripada & Rauch, 2015), which impairs understanding of the role habituation plays in long-term anxiety reduction. In summary, stay tuned on the issue of habituation; its utility in exposure therapy is not presently fully resolved. Indeed, we may someday be able to integrate aspects of the habituation model with the inhibitory learning model. As previously noted, different patients need to learn different things during exposure.

So what does Miquel learn according to the inhibitory learning model? Based off this model, when Miquel engages in exposure he is learning that the previously neutral construct of "car," which acquired an association of "danger" during the accident, now acquires a second meaning of "safety." This new safety learning then competes with the danger learning whenever Miquel encounters cars. If the safety learning is sufficiently strong, then it will inhibit the danger meaning (hence, "inhibitory learning"), and Miquel will not feel intense anxiety.

Unfortunately for us, as clinicians treating anxiety, safety learning is weaker than danger/fear learning. This makes sense from an evolutionary perspective. If you are attacked by a bear, it makes sense to rapidly acquire fear of not only the bear that attacked you but also all bears and bear-related situations that might be associated with bear attacks. You are unlikely to survive many bear attacks (you are lucky you survived the first one!), so this rapid, highly generalized, robust fear learning makes sense. If you subsequently go to Russia and have a positive experience with a tamed bear named Stephan, it would not be good to generalize that safety learning to all bears and assume all bears are safe. Instead, that safety learning should be very specific to Stephan and should only override the danger/fear learning in that very specific context.

There are a number of recommendations for how to optimize exposure, which arise from the inhibitory learning model and the associated empirical research supporting it (see Craske et al., 2008, 2014; Knowles & Olatunji, 2019, for additional discussion). A key feature that holds for many of these suggestions is the explicit recognition, as previously noted, that safety learning is weaker and very context-specific. If you keep this in mind, you will be a better exposure clinician. Note that many of the following strategies overlap in aims.

Strategies for Strengthening Safety Learning During Exposure

- Vary the context in which your patients conduct exposure.
  - If your patient only does exposure in your office, safety learning will often be constrained to your office. Your patient needs to engage in exposure in as many contexts as possible so as to generalize safety learning. Keep in mind that contexts are not only external but also internal. If your patient only learns safety while taking a particular medication and that medication is discontinued, safety learning may not generalize to the nonmedicated state. Patients who intend to

discontinue medication should optimally do so before all exposure is completed.
- To vary context in his sitting-in-a-car in vivo exposure, Miquel sat in his wife's car in many different locations, not just the clinic parking lot. He also varied the time of day.
- Vary features of the stimuli.
  - Exposure to many different types of spiders as opposed to one type of spider is more likely to produce generalized safety learning. The same is true for other fears. Predictable exposure also may serve as a context. So once your patient has some positive experiences with exposure and is engaged with the technique, instead of proceeding item by item up the graduated hierarchy, consider moving around the exposure hierarchy in a more variable, unpredictable fashion.
  - Miquel not only sat in his wife's car, he sat in his new car, in his brother's car, and in friends' cars.
  - Miquel also agreed to engaging in unpredictable exposure. His therapist gave him an envelope with pieces of paper in it. Each piece of paper listed a different car to which Miquel had access. When it was time to practice home-based exposure, Miquel would pull a car description out of the envelope and would then use that car for his exposure. So Miquel did not know which car would be used in each exposure way in advance.
- Explicitly aim to teach tolerance of anxiety instead of creating an expectation for habituation.
  - Most of your patients will benefit from being explicitly told that one aim of exposure is for them to learn to better tolerate their anxiety—even the very intense anxiety associated with panic. One common therapist mistake in treating panic is to approach treatment with the aim of having patients learn to go places without panicking. Instead, you want your patients to learn that they can shop, drive a car, watch their kids, etc. while panicking. Panic, while unpleasant, is safe and tolerable.
  - Instead of setting up the expectation that Miquel's anxiety would decrease during his first session of exposure (per the habituation model), Miquel's therapist told him that one aim of exposure is to learn that he can tolerate his anxiety.
- Also teach tolerance of uncertainty.
  - Many patients are just as intolerant of uncertainty as they are of anxiety. Exposure can be an opportunity to learn tolerance of uncertainty. Once your patient has bought into exposure and experienced some success, see if she would be willing for you to pick stimuli for exposure without telling her exactly what will happen in the next session.
  - Miquel's therapist arranged to use colleagues' cars, in addition to her own. During several sessions Miquel had no idea what type of car

would be used, if it would be running or not, or whether he would sit in the drivers sear or front passenger seat.
- Remove safety behaviors.
  - Safety behaviors and signals increase a sense of safety when avoidance of fear-provoking situations is not possible. Common safety signals/behaviors include bringing a safe person, presence of medication (even expired), cell phones, etc. Although safety behaviors may initially be needed to get your patient to engage in exposure, you should phase these out as fast as possible during therapy.
  - Miquel initially could only be in car with a safe person (e.g., his wife or therapist) but quickly progressed to sitting in the car on his own.
- Seek to maximally violate expectancies.
  - Anxiety is associated with expectations of harm (i.e., harm expectancies), and research clearly supports that notion the exposure works in part by altering these expectancies (Hofmann, 2008). Research also suggests that safety learning may be stronger when such expectancies are clearly violated. For this to happen, your patient needs to be attending to her harm expectancies. Instead of reassuring your patient that the situation is truly safe (although anxiety-provoking), have her think about her worst fear during exposure so she can clearly learn it does not actually happen. This will increase the probability that your patient alters her harm expectancy.
  - Before each exposure, Miquel articulated his worst fear. After exposure, his therapist asked him what he had learned. For instance, during his first exposure session, Miquel's biggest fear was that he would throw up, run screaming from the car, and "look like a mad man who needs to be locked up." After the exposure, he reported learning that "exposure is terrible, but it wasn't as bad as I feared. I can handle my anxiety better than I thought I would. And I stayed in the car."
- Deepen safety learning.
  - Once you have successfully conducted exposure to individual stimuli or situations, begin layering them by combining them in different combinations. For example, you can combine an interoceptive exposure exercise that your patient has mastered with going to a feared locale to which he also has successfully completed exposure. Although each situation individually no longer evokes significant fear, combining them can strengthen safety learning.
  - Miquel eventually drove different cars, listening to the feared music, all over different parts of his city.

One way to summarize these strategies is to "mix it up"—new learning needs to take place in different settings, with different features, at different times, with different stimuli. This approach is quite different to the strict following of hierarchies that often occurs in graded exposure, although we acknowledge that many of the previous strategies have been used by experienced exposure clinicians during graded exposure. If you use these suggested strategies, your patients' anxiety will be elevated, but their learning also will be wider, deeper, and more sustained. Later in this book, we detail what implications this approach has for our work with EDs (e.g., how you work with patients' fear of eating and gaining weight uncontrollably), but for now let's consider what ED clinicians can learn from the anxiety disorder field.

WHAT CAN WE LEARN FROM EXPOSURE WITH ANXIETY DISORDERS?

The use of exposure is much more common in the treatment of anxiety disorders as compared to EDs. Several lessons for ED clinicians can be gleaned from exposure for anxiety disorders.

Lessons from Anxiety Disorders

- Push beyond "normal."
  - *What anxiety clinicians typically do:* It is not uncommon for OCD therapists to have patients engage in exposure tasks (e.g., eating off the ground, wiping hands around a toilet) that make "normal" people without OCD cringe. As noted in Chapter 2, social phobia treatment frequently includes trying to invoke negative social reactions toward patients so they can be exposed to their fears of negative social evaluation.
  - *What ED clinicians typically do:* ED therapists who use exposure have a tendency to play it safe relative to anxiety disorder therapists. For instance, ED patients frequently fear negative commentary about weight, shape, or what they eat, but most ED therapists do not include exposure to such scenarios.
  - *What ED clinicians could do differently:* The anxiety disorder literature suggests we need to increase the aversiveness of exposure situations to better prepare our patients for the myriad of "real-world" stimuli they may encounter.
- Know when you are not doing exposure.
  - *What anxiety clinicians typically do:* Anxiety disorder therapists realize there are times when their patients are going to need to do something anxiety-provoking and just get through it. They also realize that it is *not* exposure *therapy* if the situation is not set up to teach anxiety tolerance and safety learning. For instance, if a panic patient has to attend an appointment and can only attend with their safe person, anxiety disorder therapists do not consider that exposure

therapy. It is possible that the patient might gain some safety learning from such an experience, but anxiety therapists do not count on this being a core element of treatment.
- *What ED clinicians typically do:* ED clinicians often view engagement in anything anxiety-provoking as exposure, even when the situation is not set up to teach anxiety tolerance or safety learning. For instance, ED clinicians frequently presume that all eating is exposure if it makes patients anxious. Involuntary eating, however, may teach neither anxiety tolerance nor safety learning; instead, the patient just "white knuckles" her way through the experience, often deploying as many safety behaviors as possible. White knuckling involves behaviorally engaging in exposure while mentally resisting the anxiety, as opposed to accepting or leaning into anxiety. Although some patients do learn anxiety tolerance and safety learning in such situations, many do not. ED clinicians also typically consider eating food while at very low weight exposure therapy, even though such a scenario may support the harm expectancy of significant weight gain. Yet, according to the inhibitory learning model, it is important to both identify and violate harm expectancies.
- *What ED clinicians could do differently:* Distinguish between eating that is primarily for the purpose of refeeding a starved body and brain versus eating that is set up to teach anxiety tolerance and safety learning. Do not presume that all involuntary eating will teach these necessary lessons.
- Provide an explicit rationale for exposure
  - *What anxiety clinicians typically do:* Anxiety disorder therapists know the importance of clearly selling the rationale for exposure therapy so that patients have good reasons to expect that treatment will work, even though it will be hard and anxiety-provoking. This will include psychoeducation that explains the link between the anxiety and treatment.
  - *What ED clinicians typically do:* In many cases ED clinicians assume that patients will intuitively grasp the rationale for exposure even though it is not explicitly laid out and sold to the patient.
  - *What ED clinicians could do differently:* Provide a clear and compelling rationale for engaging in exposure. The rationale should provide hope and elevate patient expectancies that recovery is possible, albeit challenging.

SUMMARY

Exposure is a very intuitive, albeit anxiety-provoking, intervention. Over the years, a number of models have been proposed to explain how exposure works. Although no one knows for sure exactly how exposure works, the recent inhibitory learning model offers a number of concrete and logical strategies for strengthening safety learning. Importantly, many of these strategies (e.g., varying the context of exposure and anxiety tolerance) have been clinically used by experienced exposure therapists for a long time. As such, they are backed by both the science (and logic) of the inhibitory learning model and clinical wisdom.

4

Why Exposure for Eating Disorders?

A Rationale for Treatment

Now that we have reviewed how exposure therapy is used to address a variety of anxiety-related problems, we turn our attention to the rationale for applying this treatment to eating disorders (EDs). You will benefit from having a thorough understanding of this rationale in two key ways. First, you will likely experience a greater sense of confidence in your ability to conceptualize and treat a variety of ED cases from an exposure-based framework. Rather than worrying about establishing the "correct diagnosis" for your patient and/or choosing the treatment manual/guide that pertains to that diagnosis, you will understand how exposure-based strategies apply to key transdiagnostic features that underpin many EDs (e.g., Murray et al., 2018). Second, you will be able to convey your understanding to your patients so that they can understand why exposure is a good "fit" with ED treatment. This can increase your patients' investment in the treatment and optimism about a positive outcome—both of which are associated with good response to treatment. Accordingly, this chapter provides you with an overview of three critical reasons why exposure ought to be a tool you employ consistently in your work with individuals with EDs.

REASON #1: CONTENT OVERLAP

Put simply, the overlap in content between EDs and anxiety disorders is significant. Indeed, several defensible arguments have been made to conceptualize EDs as a variant of a larger, encompassing anxiety "syndrome" (e.g., Waller, 2008). So extensive is the conceptual and phenomenological overlap between EDs and anxiety disorders that it is beyond the scope of this chapter to review it comprehensively. As such, what follows are descriptions of what we believe to be the four most critical shared features between EDs and anxiety disorders: (a) preoccupation with feared outcomes, (b) avoidance of distressing stimuli, (c) safety behaviors, and (d) the functional relatedness of the preceding symptoms. Having a firm grasp of these features will help you better to "see" EDs through the lens of empirically supported models of how anxiety disorders manifest and persist. This understanding is essential to your effective application of exposure with EDs.

Preoccupation with Feared Outcomes

Individuals suffering from anxiety disorders experience persistent preoccupation with a vast array of feared outcomes. From acquiring a fatal illness to being publicly humiliated, the range of possibilities of feared outcomes is essentially limitless. Many feared outcomes involve consequences that are unquestionably catastrophic (e.g., being responsible for the death of a child). Often, the driving force behind these types of fears is the tendency to overestimate the *likelihood* of such catastrophic outcomes (e.g., Salkovskis et al., 2000). By comparison, other feared outcomes are less severe (e.g., losing one's wallet). Nonetheless, the perceived threat of these outcomes causes intense fear for certain individuals because of their tendency to overestimate the *cost* of such outcomes. That is, individuals who experience pathological anxiety often believe that relatively common mishaps would be unbearably distressing (Wilson & Rapee, 2005). For example, missing a bus (low threat) will be accompanied by thoughts of arriving late at work, failing in a key task as a result, and being fired (high cost). The tendency to overestimate the likelihood and/or severity of negative consequences is a critical driver of fear preoccupation (Clark, 1999). Indeed, many established measurements of anxiety disorder symptom severity assess the extent to which individuals report being preoccupied with feared outcomes (e.g., Steketee, Frost, & Bogart, 1996), indicating the transdiagnostic relevance of this construct across anxiety disorders.

Your ED patients will be just as preoccupied with feared outcomes. Indeed, an increasing body of research has converged on the finding that across ED diagnoses, concern with feared outcomes related to eating is central to ED pathology (Levinson et al., 2017; Murray et al., 2018; Smith et al., 2018). Common examples of feared outcomes in EDs include continuous, exorbitant weight gain, inability to tolerate even low to moderate amounts of "surplus" weight, inability to tolerate anxiety while eating, and losing control over eating. Other less typical feared outcomes in EDs that nonetheless present occasionally (particularly with avoidant/restrictive food intake disorder [ARFID]) include choking or vomiting uncontrollably while eating, experiencing unbearable disgust over the texture of certain foods, and suffering a serious medical consequence as a result of one's eating habits (e.g., developing heart disease from nominal consumption of butter).

Similar to anxiety disorders, your patient's preoccupation with feared outcomes in EDs will stem from overestimations of the likelihood and/or severity of potential threats. To illustrate, it is very common for individuals with EDs to overestimate the influence that normative dietary intake will have on weight gain (Waller

& Mountford, 2015). More specifically, they believe it is very likely that they will gain a significant amount of weight with normal eating. Similarly, individuals with ARFID who have experienced or witnessed choking on food in the past tend to overestimate the likelihood that this will occur again.

EDs also often involve substantial overestimation of the cost (i.e., severity) of outcomes that are fairly common if not unavoidable. For instance, adolescents with EDs often fear that changes to weight and body shape, as part of pubertal development, will be overwhelming and intolerable. Similarly, for someone with an ED, eating 10 kcal more than "allowed" might be a low threat in an objective sense, but their exaggerated belief in the consequences (e.g., ballooning in weight and losing all friends as a result) makes for a very high potential cost. Not surprisingly, research indicates that the frequency and intensity of preoccupation with feared outcomes is high in both EDs and anxiety disorders, with no significant differences between the two (García-Soriano, Roncero, Perpiñá, & Belloch, 2014).

Avoidance of Distressing Stimuli

In response to their preoccupation with feared outcomes, many individuals with anxiety disorders engage in a predictable pattern of avoiding stimuli that they associate with feared outcomes. Just as the range of fears is limitless, so is the range of things that anxious individuals avoid. These avoidant tendencies serve two chief functions for individuals with anxiety disorders. First, they preclude any encounter with a stimulus assumed to be threatening, thereby minimizing the likelihood of harm, as Janet's case illustrates.

> Janet feared that entering an oncology clinic would cause her to develop cancer. Not surprisingly, Janet avoided going into, or near, oncology clinics as well as related stimuli. For instance, Janet avoided doctors. She was particularly afraid of oncology doctors but also avoided other doctors because they might have come in contact with oncology doctors either via work ("They all go to hospitals at some point") or by socializing ("Doctors probably hang around other doctors").

The second major function of avoidant behaviors is to prevent or escape negative emotional experiences that an individual, such as Joshua, believes to be overwhelming or intolerable.

> Joshua was afraid of attending temple because he feared being unable to tolerate the anxiety he experienced secondary to doubts over whether or not he was a "true believer" of the Jewish faith. Joshua's children attended a Jewish school, and he avoided picking them up or attending parent–teacher

> meetings for the same reason. Joshua also feared that the teachers would detect his "religious flaws" even on the phone, so he made his wife handle all teacher discussions.

Lastly, it is important to point out that not all forms of avoidance are directly observable (i.e., noticeable). Many anxious patients engage in patterns of cognitive avoidance that are more subtle and thus difficult to detect. Perhaps the most notable example of this is the avoidance of trauma-related cognitions (i.e., memories) that is characteristic of individuals with PTSD

If you have worked with individuals with EDs, you have undoubtedly noticed many similar avoidant tendencies. Similar to anxiety disorders, there is a wide array of scenarios and stimuli that individuals with EDs avoid. In many cases, the avoidant behaviors serve the purpose of trying to prevent a feared outcome. Selective food avoidance is a common feature across EDs and is often intended as a means to prevent anticipated weight gain. Indeed, it is most often the highly palatable, calorically dense foods (e.g., pastries) that individuals with EDs such as A'isha "ban" from their diet (Marzola, Nasser, Hashim, Shih, & Kaye, 2013).

> A'isha reported eating a very limited diet of egg whites, grilled chicken, pickles, salad greens sprinkled with vinegar, and, occasionally, dry wheat toast. She reported that she had not eaten cheese, ice cream, butter, hamburgers, French fries, cake, cookies, or any oil in three years. She reported believing that consuming even a small amount of these foods would lead her to "blow up like a balloon." Although she loved lattes, she only drank unsweetened black coffee so she could "see that nothing else had slipped into it."

For an additional example of trying to avoid a feared outcome that is different from "classic" ED body image disturbances, consider the case of Christopher.

> Christopher witnessed his aunt choke while eating and subsequently developed an intense fear of choking. Christopher avoided taking normal-sized bites of food and chewed each bite of food for an extended period of time before swallowing. He also ate at a very slow pace and preferred "wet" or "slippery" foods that were less likely to cause him to choke.

There are also a number of common avoidance behaviors in EDs that together share the core function of escaping from aversive emotional states that are perceived to be unbearable. As noted by Waller and Mountford (2015), many ED patients believe they are not capable of tolerating the emotional distress around learning their weight and subsequently avoid scenarios in which they would become aware of their weight.

> Jordan, a transgender person, had lost significant weight over the past two years but feared they might gain it back. Jordan was very anxious about their weight and refused to be weighed. They would not step on a scale at home and refused to be weighed at medical appointments because they were certain that they would "totally melt down" if they found out they had gained any weight. Maintaining an appearance of "having my act together" was very important to Jordan, which made the idea of "melting down" particularly unacceptable.

Related to weight avoidance, many individuals with EDs engage in a broader assortment of body image avoidance behaviors. Together, these behaviors serve the function of suppressing negative emotional experiences related to body image. Common examples of these behaviors include avoiding clothing items that are "revealing" of one's physique and avoiding certain activities that one associates with body image-related scrutiny (Rosen, Srebnik, Saltzberg, & Wendt, 1991).

> Jordan also avoided exercising in a crowded gym, preferring to go at odd hours when it was most likely to be quiet or even empty. In addition, Jordan stayed away from people who evoked perceptions of body image-related inferiority. For instance, they stopped hanging out with a friend who "had a much better body." Jordan also bowed out of conversations in which weight and/or body shape might become the central topic of discussion.

Finally, although binge eating is often an unintended consequence of restrictive eating, binge eating also can occur secondary to cognitive avoidance of negative emotions. Heatherton and Baumeister (1991) were among the first to propose that when individuals become aware of disliked aspects of themselves and experience negative emotions, they may engage in cognitive avoidance (i.e., escape from their self-awareness). This cognitive avoidance, in turn, leaves them susceptible to impulsive behaviors, such as binge eating. If this occurs repeatedly, individuals learn that binge eating reduces the intensity of their negative emotions, and binge eating becomes negatively reinforced. Additionally, binge eating can be involved in more than just avoidance of negative cognitions and emotions. Many individuals with EDs describe patterns of binge eating that occur in the immediate aftermath of interpersonal conflict (e.g., Luo, Nuttall, Locke, & Hopwood, 2018).

Safety Behaviors

Chapters 1 and 2 made occasional reference to safety behaviors, which we define here as actions taken with the aim of detecting and neutralizing potentially threatening scenarios or stimuli. You will see that A'isha is using a range of such behaviors (checking on her grandmother's cooking; checking restaurant menus to confirm calorie counts; checking her body).

> A'isha weighed herself excessively (e.g., after each time she ate) and also repeatedly checked the appearance of her physique in the mirror to gauge for possible increases in her weight or body size. She reported she was able to "breathe a sigh of relief" if everything seemed the same. In addition, A'isha carefully watched how her grandmother prepared food when she visited to make sure she didn't add any extra fat or sugar. She noted that her grandmother understood she was on a very limited diet, but she just needed to make sure her grandmother didn't accidentally "slip up" for her own peace of mind. She also extensively researched nutritional information if she was forced to eat at a restaurant, so that she could make sure she stayed within a "reasonable" calorie limit and relax enough to "pretend to be normal."

In the field of anxiety disorders, it is well-established that safety behaviors play a crucial role in the development and maintenance of pathological anxiety. There are several important reasons why this is so. First, safety behaviors are temporarily "effective" in relieving distress and, thus, are negatively reinforced. Additionally, safety behaviors function similarly to avoidance (see previous section), in that they prevent individuals from having experiences that would otherwise disconfirm their anticipatory feared outcomes. Related to this, when your patient encounters a feared scenario, engages in safety behaviors, and observes that her feared outcome does not occur, it is likely that she will attribute the nonoccurrence of her feared outcome to her safety behaviors (Salkovskis, 1991). That is, safety behaviors are perceived by the individual as the only thing that prevented what was otherwise an assured negative outcome. For instance, after having to eat out several times in one week, A'isha noted that she would have "definitely gained weight" if not for her research.

Similar to avoidance of distressing stimuli, the use of safety behaviors is pervasive in individuals with EDs. Table 4.1 provides a list of safety/avoidant behaviors that are frequently used in EDs, as well as the common functions that these behaviors serve. Some of these behaviors are broadly aimed at detecting potentially threatening outcomes, such as A'isha's frequent weight and body checking. Other ED safety behaviors are more directly intended to prevent an anticipated negative outcome from occurring. Purging behaviors and compulsive exercising are two characteristic ways that individuals who are fearful of weight gain attempt to keep themselves from gaining weight.

It also is common for individuals with EDs to engage in a variety of eating-related safety behaviors to reduce anxiety around eating (Gianini et al., 2015). Common examples of these (often bizarre) eating-related safety behaviors include eating at an exceedingly slow pace, taking only very small bites of food, mixing foods together that are not typically combined, and excessive manipulation of food prior to eating (e.g., using napkins to absorb oil or butter from the surface of

Table 4.1. COMMON SAFETY/AVOIDANT BEHAVIORS IN EATING DISORDERS AND THEIR TYPICAL FUNCTION(S)

Safety/Avoidant Behavior	Typical Function of Behavior	Chapters Referenced
Caloric restriction	Limit caloric intake to prevent weight gain	10, 12, 13
Body/weight checking	Detect potential changes in weight and/or body shape	10, 12, 13
Compulsive exercise	Burn calories to prevent weight gain; modify body physique	10, 12
Self-induced vomiting	Limit caloric intake to prevent weight gain	10, 12, 13
Using laxatives/diuretics	Limit caloric intake to prevent weight gain	10, 12, 13
Wearing baggy clothing	Concealing body size/shape from others	13
Food-related research	Gain awareness of the caloric content or nutritional value of foods	10
Eating very slowly	Prevent loss of control over eating; achieve satiation before finishing	10, 14, 15
Eating very quickly	Escape negative emotions that accompany eating	10, 14
Ripping/tearing food	Prevent loss of control over eating; slow the pace of eating	10
Odd food mixtures	Limit enjoyment of food by making it unpalatable	10
Taking very small bites	Prevent loss of control over eating; prevent choking on food	10, 14, 15
Manipulating food	Limit caloric intake to prevent weight gain	10
Overdressing	Overheat to induce sweating and lose weight	15
Underdressing	Cause body shivering to burn calories	15
Adjusting body posture	Mitigate distressing physiological arousal; control body appearance	13, 15
Comparing self to others	Assess "acceptability" of one's physique compared to that of others	13
Seeking reassurance	Neutralize uncertainty about food content and/or body image	10, 12, 13, 14

food). It is important to note, as Vitousek (2019) has explained, that some of these behaviors can, at times, be a normative response to starvation in very low-weight patients. For instance, slow eating *may* serve as a mechanism to reduce consumption. However, it also may be a relatively automatic savoring behavior associated with starvation in people who want to eat. Similarly, creation of odd combinations of food has been observed in people who are starved for reasons other than an ED (Tucker, 2006). In contrast, using napkins to absorb oil is quite specific to EDs.

The complexity of behaviors that can serve as safety behaviors highlights the need to engage in careful functional assessment to determine the purpose of any given behavior (Murray et al., 2016) or to develop hypotheses about what that purpose might be. We discuss this further in Chapter 6, but as an immediate example, blotting oil from the surface of food secondary to texture-related disgust/anxiety serves a very different purpose compared to when it is done to reduce calories. As you will see in later chapters, exposure to address the core pathology might look very different based on the different functions potentially associated with any one behavior.

Functional Relatedness of Symptoms

Finally, in addition to EDs and anxiety disorders having a great deal of overlap with regard to symptom content, they also share a commonality regarding the functional relatedness of these symptoms. In other words, the patterns of interaction between individuals' feared concerns and behavioral responses (i.e., avoidance and safety behaviors) in EDs and anxiety tend to mirror one another. In the case of anxiety disorders, preoccupation with feared outcomes and subsequent avoidance/safety behaviors are typically functionally related to one another, and their consistent pairing leads to them becoming increasingly associated with (and predictive of) one another (Abramowitz, Taylor, & McKay, 2009). For example, an individual who is fearful of contracting serious illness from contact with common objects or surfaces may compulsively wash his hands whenever he touches a feared object or surface. His engagement in the handwashing safety behavior will contribute to more intense preoccupation with his feared outcomes, which, in turn, will instigate further handwashing.

This reciprocal influence between preoccupation with feared outcomes and engagement in avoidance/safety behaviors is also frequently observed in EDs. For instance, among individuals with EDs, distinctive patterns of preoccupation with feared outcomes (e.g., experiencing noticeable changes to body size) are prospectively predictive of specific safety behaviors (e.g., body checking), and vice versa (Levinson et al., 2018). Thus, it appears a similar interactive feedback loop between feared concerns and avoidance/safety behaviors that is a hallmark of OCD and other anxiety problems is also present in EDs. This is especially important in the context of EDs, given recent work showing that reductions in patients' preoccupation with feared outcomes *and* safety behaviors during the course of treatment are both prospectively predictive of global ED treatment outcome (Farrell, Brosof, et al., 2019).

REASON #2: COMORBIDITY

In addition to the overlap in symptom content between EDs and anxiety disorders, there is also substantial comorbidity between the two. A wealth of research demonstrates this comorbidity, with the general pattern of findings indicating that well over half of individuals with EDs experience clinical symptoms of at least one anxiety condition (Kaye, Bulik, Thornton, Barbarich, & Masters, 2004). Some of the most commonly co-occurring anxiety conditions include OCD, social anxiety disorder, and PTSD (Kaye et al., 2004). Unfortunately, there is robust evidence indicating that the presence of comorbid clinical anxiety symptoms confers risk for suboptimal ED treatment outcome (Vall & Wade, 2015). Although the reasons for this are unclear, it has been suggested that engaging in an ED may be one way that individuals regulate the intense distress they experience associated with their anxiety condition. An important finding supporting this theory is that anxiety disorders tend to predate the onset of ED symptoms in most patients (Swinbourne & Touyz, 2007).

At this point, you might be discouraged and asking yourself if there is any hope for your ED patients. After all, if the majority of them are likely experiencing comorbid anxiety disorders, which can act as a barrier to optimal treatment response, how can one muster any hope? Fortunately, there is empirical evidence showing that exposure-based therapy applied simultaneously to EDs and comorbid anxiety problems can be helpful in reducing symptoms of both co-occurring conditions (Simpson et al., 2013). The elevated likelihood of encountering comorbid anxiety problems when working with ED patients is further rationale for ED clinicians to utilize exposure therapy routinely in their practice. From your patient's point of view, it may be a more feasible proposition to adhere to one set of core treatment guidelines (e.g., confront your feared situations and disengage from safety behaviors and avoidance) rather than trying to juggle multiple disorder-specific treatment protocols at the same time. Lastly, using an exposure-based approach to address your patient's ED and anxiety disorder may provide opportunity for "layering" different exposure stimuli in the same therapeutic exercise to achieve deepened extinction learning (Culver, Vervliet, & Craske, 2014). We discuss this in detail provide examples throughout the book.

REASON #3: MANY EVIDENCE-BASED TREATMENTS ARE INHERENTLY EXPOSURE-BASED

There are several treatment protocols that have demonstrated a solid evidence base in the treatment of EDs. Of note, CBT and family-based treatment (FBT) have amassed the greatest degree of empirical support, with dozens of studies attesting to the efficacy of these treatments. Although both contain a variety of different strategies, it can be argued that the key "active ingredients" of each are inherently exposure-based. The same can also be argued for some other evidence-based therapies—particularly specialist supportive clinical management for AN.

To illustrate, in evidence-based CBT for EDs, patients are encouraged to confront their anxiety around weight and body shape via weekly weighing sessions in which patients are told their weight. This weighing procedure also allows patients the opportunity to disconfirm their expectations of exorbitant weight gain (Waller & Mountford, 2015). Additionally, patients receiving CBT are encouraged to gradually include feared/avoided foods into their diet with increasing regularity over the course of treatment (Fairburn, 2008). Finally, body image-focused exposure (see Chapter 13) can be included as a key component of CBT for EDs. Although CBT contains other nonexposure components, such as cognitive therapy strategies to address the maladaptive cognitions and emotional aspects of EDs, there is evidence to suggest that the exposure-based aspects of CBT are principally responsible for the overall therapeutic benefit (Waller & Raykos, 2019).

The specific mechanisms of action in FBT are unclear. However, it is plausible that the efficacy of FBT is driven, at least in part, by intensive feeding exposure in which food is eaten more frequently, in larger quantities, and with foods that were previously avoided (Hildebrandt, Bacow, Markella, & Loeb, 2012). Moreover, because the treatment is conducted almost entirely in the individual's natural (i.e., home) environment, as opposed to a clinic or hospital, the learning that takes place in feeding exposure likely generalizes to a greater extent. FBT also explicitly targets safety behaviors and particularly aims to eliminate those that interfere with achievement of improved nutritional stability (e.g., compulsive exercising, purging). Of course, it is important to stress to your patient that all such work needs to be structured to be a learning experience—not just eating and white knuckling the anxiety. Finally, similar to CBT, FBT includes regular exposure to weight on a weekly basis, which likely yields reductions in fear about weight gain.

Aside from CBT and FBT, other ED treatment approaches that are implemented by a wide range of providers (e.g., dietitians, psychologists, physicians, nurses etc.) share the same key objectives of guiding patients in normalization of dietary intake and cessation of unhealthy safety behaviors. Because many ED patients are, at a minimum, reluctant to cooperate with these recommended changes, we contend that an exposure-based approach to these changes represents one of the most practical and achievable courses of action for two primary reasons. First, reluctance to begin confronting feared stimuli and to stop safety behaviors is characteristic of anxiety disorders. In most cases, however, individuals with anxiety disorders can be brought tentatively on board by starting with small changes before graduating to the more wholesale changes that result in the elimination of their pathological fear and avoidance. This mirrors our experience in applying exposure to EDs: most patients are only willing to go along with minor changes at first but become increasingly willing to engage in more significant change as their confidence grows. Second, exposure therapy is a very collaborative treatment, which offers patients a reasonably high degree of agency in decision-making with regard to selecting targets for exposure as well as the pace of treatment. As such, we find exposure to be a useful means of navigating through the typical hesitancy that many ED patients initially bring to the table (pun intended).

SUMMARY

In this chapter, we have outlined a theoretically based rationale for using exposure consistently in the treatment of individuals with EDs. Due to the substantial overlap between EDs and anxiety disorders (both in symptom content and in comorbidity between the conditions), exposure therapy is a sound choice for therapeutic intervention. Indeed, the most evidence-based treatments for EDs contain a number of exposure-based strategies that drive much of the therapeutic benefit. Of course, the rationale for using exposure that we have outlined in this chapter means very little if there are no data that provide empirical support for exposure in treatment of EDs. In Chapter 5, we will comprehensively review the extant research that supports exposure as an effective approach for EDs.

5

How Well Does Exposure Therapy Work for Eating Disorders?

A Summary of the Evidence

In Chapter 3, we provided an overview of the theoretically based mechanisms of change in exposure therapy. Hopefully, that overview helped you to develop a solid understanding of how exposure therapy exerts its therapeutic influence in individuals who struggle with intense anxiety and who cope ineffectively through avoidance and safety behaviors. You should now have a good understanding of key exposure principles like violation of fear expectancies and habituation. However, having a knowledge of how exposure therapy theoretically works is not sufficient by itself. What you will need in addition to this is a thorough understanding of how *well* exposure therapy works in relieving the symptoms of individuals with EDs. An ability to convey this understanding to your patients in relatively simple, understandable language can go a long way toward increasing their confidence in the treatment.

If you are reading this and asking yourself, "Exposure sounds like it could work, but will it actually help my ED patients?" you may not be alone. Compared to the very well-established evidence base for exposure therapy across anxiety disorders, there has been substantially less investigation of the effects of exposure applied to EDs. However, it is important to remember that exposure (even when not formally labeled as such) is present to some degree in all evidence-based treatments for EDs (Becker & Waller, 2017). Unfortunately, research that supports packaged treatments (such as CBT or FBT) does not provide information on which elements of the treatment are most critical. Moreover, as discussed further in Chapter 9, some components of standard evidence-based treatment may or may not be exposure, depending on exactly how the clinician uses the clinical strategy. Thus, we still need studies that specifically focus on identifying the benefits of exposure for EDs. Fortunately, there is a growing body of literature attesting to the benefits of exposure therapy in treating individuals with EDs. Although rather heterogeneous, much of this literature can be categorized into one of three separate domains: (a) food exposure to address eating-related fears, (b) body-focused exposure to address body image-related anxiety, and (c) cue exposure to address binge eating. In this chapter, we will review and summarize the empirical evidence for exposure therapy within each of these three domains. We start by considering the case of Bruno, whose symptoms present the opportunity to implement each of these three types of exposure in his treatment.

> Bruno is a 25-year-old man with a history of body image disturbance that dates back to his teenage years, when he was a competitive gymnast. During this period of his life, Bruno perceived strong pressure to have a very lean and muscular build, and he grew steadily more preoccupied with trying to modify his body accordingly. He began engaging in frequent body checking and compulsive muscle-tensing behaviors in response to fear that his body was not ideally "trim and toned."
>
> In relation to his increased body image anxiety, Bruno developed restrictive eating habits that involved decreasing the overall quantity of food he consumed as well as cutting many "junk foods" (e.g., desserts, fried foods, and other calorie-dense foods) out of his diet. This restraint in his eating caused him to lose weight and temporarily feel a sense of satisfaction. However, his anxiety about body size and shape quickly returned, which further fueled his patterns of restrictive eating habits, body checking, and compulsive physical exertion.
>
> Bruno's restrictive diet was insufficient to meet his body's energy needs and contributed to uncontrollable episodes of bingeing on many of the foods that he desperately tried to avoid. These binge-eating episodes quickly became more frequent and typically were triggered by negative mood states. To illustrate, on one occasion when he was angry after receiving a driving citation, he rapidly ate an entire cake that his roommate had baked for a birthday party. Bruno's bingeing led to steady weight gain and increased body image anxiety. He subsequently became very avoidant of situations and other stimuli (e.g., wearing a swimsuit) that provoked body image anxiety.

FOOD EXPOSURE

Like many individuals with EDs, Bruno experienced intense fear of consuming larger quantities of food as well as specific food items. Whereas the most common feared outcome related to food consumption is significant, uncontrollable weight gain, some patients' eating-related fears include medical catastrophes, severe choking and/or vomiting, or encountering unbearable disgust associated with aversive tastes or textures of food. These eating-related fears account for much of the heightened degree of food avoidance and overall dietary inflexibility in EDs, and, as such, they are important targets for exposure intervention.

Fears of uncontrollable weight gain and other eating fears can be addressed effectively with food-based exposure. In this approach, the clinician and patient collaboratively implement exposure tasks to systematically confront feared and avoided scenarios, such as eating sufficient quantities of food to maintain or increase weight and introducing "forbidden" foods into the patient's diet. Other common exposure themes include eating in the presence of other people, eating in unfamiliar and unpredictable settings (e.g., trying a new restaurant), and breaking long-held rules about when, how, and why food is eaten (e.g., no eating after 8:00 PM; must be last person at the table to finish food, etc.). The clinician and patient also work together to identify and reduce safety behaviors used by the patient to neutralize anxiety around eating (e.g., tearing food into small pieces) or directly prevent feared outcomes (e.g., chewing food excessively before swallowing to prevent choking). Chapter 10 provides a more in-depth description of how food exposure is implemented.

Single Case Studies

A handful of single case studies provided preliminary evidence for the effectiveness of food exposure. In one of the first documented investigations, Mavissakalian (1982) described the use of food exposure paired with prevention of compulsive exercising for two adolescent females. Although both patients were markedly underweight at treatment baseline and experiencing other associated medical issues, they gained weight appropriately and showed reductions in anxiety during eating, per the observation of the experimenters. Another case report described the implementation of food exposure, in which an adult male patient with extreme eating anxiety and avoidance successfully incorporated a variety of "forbidden" foods into his diet, resulting in significantly decreased eating anxiety, improved tolerance of fullness sensations, and restoration of a healthy body weight (Boutelle, 1998). A more recent case study detailed the treatment of a young female patient who was guided in exposure to feared food items and prevention of eating-related safety behaviors, such as tearing up food and body checking after eating (Glasofer, Albano, Simpson, & Steinglass, 2016). Upon completion of 12 sessions of food exposure, this patient reported decreased eating anxiety, less preoccupation with food concerns, and increased caloric intake during a test meal (i.e., behavioral approach task).

Case Series

Further evidence of the benefits of food exposure has come from several case series studies in various naturalistic treatment settings. Steinglass et al. (2012) developed a 12-session food exposure therapy intervention that was used with nine patients with AN who had recently completed a course of weight restoration in an inpatient hospital setting. The patients in this study experienced decreased fear both at the outset of and during eating, which was prospectively predictive of increased food intake over the course of a week. Results from a more recent case series suggest that clinicians need not wait to begin food exposure until a patient has fully completed weight restoration. In a severe sample of over 100 ED patients requiring inpatient hospitalization, food exposure was well-tolerated by patients and resulted in reduced eating-related fears and avoidance behaviors (Farrell, Bowie, et al., 2019). Additional case series designs have shown food-based exposure therapy to be beneficial in decreasing anxiety around eating and improving nutritional stability in residential (Simpson et al., 2013) and partial hospitalization programs (Levinson & Byrne, 2015). This evidence base does not extend to younger people, given the focus on FBT rather than CBT for EDs in that age range to date, although there is no reason to assume that the same benefits would not apply.

Controlled Trials

There have also been several controlled trials that have added to the evidence base for food-based exposure. Using a randomized controlled design, Steinglass et al. (2014) compared exposure therapy with cognitive remediation therapy (CRT). They found that patients who received exposure showed significantly greater caloric intake from pretreatment to posttreatment, using a test meal. While increased caloric intake was significantly correlated with reduced eating-related fear in patients who received exposure, this relationship was not found in patients who received CRT. It is important to note, however, that while exposure was significantly better than the CRT statistically, the overall effect of exposure in this trial was clinically modest.

Two other controlled studies assessed whether exposure therapy for AN could be augmented with D-cycloserine (DCS), a pharmacological agent that has appeared promising in augmenting exposure therapy for anxiety disorders. Consistent with the literature for some other disorders (e.g., PTSD; Abdallah et al., 2019), results regarding the additional benefit of DCS have been mixed. The results of one of the ED studies indicated that DCS did not effectively augment exposure (Steinglass et al., 2007). In contrast, the other study showed that those patients who received DCS evidenced superior weight restoration (Levinson et al., 2015). Importantly, all patients in these two DCS studies were treated with food exposure therapy and experienced significant reductions in anxiety about eating.

BODY-FOCUSED EXPOSURE

At the heart of Bruno's difficulty with his ED was substantial anxiety about his body weight and shape. This anxiety manifested in compulsive body checking as well as avoidance of various things that were upsetting to him due to perceiving his body as unattractive. As an ED clinician, you will encounter many patients who share Bruno's struggle to accept the size and shape of his body. Indeed, there is a large body of literature attesting to the central role of body image disturbance in the development and maintenance of EDs (e.g., Rohde, Stice, & Marti, 2015), as well as in the re-emergence of symptoms after an initial remission (Keel, Dorer, Franko, Jackson, & Herzog, 2005).

Body-focused exposure addresses this disturbance by encouraging individuals to confront stimuli that they commonly avoid because of anxiety around their body image. To illustrate, mirror exposure is an effective and commonly used exposure technique and involves guiding patients to view their bodies in a mirror as a whole and/or moving systematically through various parts of the body (Griffen, Naumann, & Hildebrandt, 2018). Other body-focused exposure strategies involve encouraging patients to approach scenarios that are typically avoided due to body image anxiety, such as wearing form-fitting clothing (e.g., swimsuit), engaging in social activities (e.g., exercising in public), and various types of physical intimacy (Cash, 1997). Patients also are encouraged to resist engaging in safety behaviors aimed at minimizing distress around their appearance (e.g., body checking). It has been speculated that body-focused exposure exerts its therapeutic influence in one or more of the following ways: habituation of body-related anxiety (Vocks, Wächter, Wucherer, & Kosfelder, 2008), disconfirming overestimations of body size (Rushford & Ostermeyer, 1997), improved tolerance of disliked aspects of one's body (Vocks, Legenbauer, Wächter, Wucherer, & Kosfelder, 2007), and enhanced emphasis on positive aspects of one's body image (Jansen, Voorwinde, et al., 2016). The implementation of body image exposure is described in more detail in Chapter 13.

Clinical Evidence Regarding Body Exposure in Isolation

Empirical evidence supporting the use of body-focused exposure includes a number of studies in which body exposure techniques were implemented in standalone fashion, yielding change in a variety of outcome variables. The first study of this sort was done using mirror exposure to successfully reduce overestimations of body size in 24 individuals with AN or BN (Norris, 1984). The study also found that greater reductions in body size overestimation were predictive of decreased global ED pathology.

More recent studies have utilized mirror exposure combined with body exposure to other stimuli that typically evoke body image anxiety (e.g., "revealing" clothing items). These studies have demonstrated improvements in a range of outcome variables among larger, mixed-diagnosis ED samples. These improvements include a significantly reduced level of body image anxiety, evident both at the level of psychological self-report (Fernández & Vandereycken, 1994; Vocks et al., 2007) and physiological indices of anxiety (e.g., salivary cortisol levels; Díaz-Ferrer, Rodríguez-Ruiz, Ortega Roldán, Moreno-Domínguez, & Fernández-Santaella, 2015; Trentowska, Svaldi, Blechert, & Tuschen-Caffier, 2017).

Other improvements observed in studies employing body-focused exposure with clinical ED samples include decreased fears of weight gain (Rushford & Ostermeyer, 1997), reduced body-checking behavior (Vocks, Kosfelder, Wucherer, & Wächter, 2008), and diminished overvaluation of body shape and weight (Trentowska, Svaldi, & Tuschen-Caffier, 2014). The last of these addresses a central feature across EDs. It is worth noting that body-focused exposure delivered as a stand-alone intervention has yielded similar patterns of benefit among samples of larger-bodied individuals with binge-eating difficulties (Hilbert & Tuschen-Caffier, 2004; Hilbert, Tuschen-Caffier, & Vögele, 2002).

Effectiveness of Body Exposure as an Element of Other Therapies

In addition to the previously cited literature on the effects of body-focused exposure as a stand-alone therapeutic intervention, there is research demonstrating its benefits when included in several CBT protocols for clinical ED samples. In a sample of adult inpatients, Key et al. (2002) showed that a traditional CBT intervention augmented with mirror exposure was superior to traditional CBT alone in reducing body image dissatisfaction and anxiety, as well as behavioral avoidance surrounding body image. Another study showed that, as an adjunct to traditional CBT, a mirror exposure-based intervention yielded greater reductions in body-related anxiety and body-checking frequency when compared to a nondirective body image treatment (Hildebrandt, Loeb, Troupe, & Delinsky, 2012). A similar study found that among a sample of patients who had experienced partial remission of their ED symptoms in an intensive day treatment program, patients who were randomized to receive an adjunctive body-focused exposure intervention evidenced significantly greater reductions in overvaluation of body shape and weight as well as body image avoidance, compared to patients who received a treatment-as-usual maintenance intervention (Trottier, Carter, MacDonald, McFarlane, & Olmsted, 2015). Finally, several investigations of novel CBT interventions that contain a relatively high "dosage" of body-focused exposure have yielded significantly reduced body image anxiety and body-related safety behaviors (Morgan, Lazarova, Schelhase, & Saeidi, 2014; Vocks et al., 2011).

CUE EXPOSURE

Similar to many individuals who attempt to maintain a prolonged pattern of dietary restraint, Bruno experienced a breakdown in this control, succumbing to recurrent episodes of binge eating. By virtue of being frequently paired with his binge-eating episodes, various environmental stimuli (e.g., negative moods) became "conditioned" to elicit Bruno's binge-eating cravings. This exemplifies Jansen et al.'s (1989) empirically supported classical conditioning model of binge eating, which postulates that binge-eating episodes are often cued by conditioned stimuli that have repeatedly preceded binges. Common examples of conditioned stimuli that cue binge eating include various food-related interactions, such as seeing, smelling, or tasting food, as well as negative emotional experiences (Bongers & Jansen, 2017). In cue exposure, patients are guided in pairing these binge-eating cues with the *absence* of any actual binge eating, which ultimately weakens the intensity of the binge cravings. In Bruno's case, cue exposure would likely involve deliberate exposure to negative emotional experiences paired with subsequent prevention of any bingeing. We provide a more thorough description of how to implement cue exposure in Chapter 11.

Initial Studies of Cue Exposure

Initial evidence for the beneficial impact of cue exposure was provided by single case studies of patients with BN, which demonstrated that cue exposure was helpful in reducing binge-eating frequency as well as use of compensatory behaviors (Jansen et al., 1989). Additionally, a small trial found that cue exposure was superior to self-control training in reducing binge eating (Jansen, Broekmate, & Heymans, 1992). Although this study only included six patients in each treatment condition, it is notable that all six patients who received cue exposure were in full remission from binge-eating symptoms at a 1-year follow-up, as compared to only two of the six patients who received self-control training. Finally, a study of a mixed-diagnosis sample of 20 ED inpatients revealed that cue exposure led to significant reductions in binge eating, purging behaviors, guilt surrounding eating, and depressive symptom severity (Kennedy, Katz, Neitzert, Ralevski, & Mendlowitz, 1995).

Controlled Studies

A few studies have examined cue exposure as either a comparison treatment to traditional CBT or as an adjunctive component of it. In a trial comparing cue exposure to CBT among 30 patients with BN, Cooper and Steere (1995) found the treatments to be equally effective in reducing binge-eating and purging frequency, although gains were better maintained in the CBT group at a 1-year follow-up. Other research has assessed the utility of cue exposure as a supplement to traditional CBT. A large randomized controlled trial including 135 patients with BN found that after a traditional course of CBT, patients who received a cue exposure intervention showed less dietary restraint, purging, body image dissatisfaction, and anxiety related to binge cues when compared to a relaxation training condition (Bulik, Sullivan, Carter, McIntosh, & Joyce, 1998). The durability of the findings from this trial was noteworthy. After 1 year, patients who received cue exposure evidenced significantly less bulimic symptoms and better overall functioning. Furthermore, these benefits remained robust at both a 3-year (Carter, McIntosh, Joyce, Sullivan, & Bulik, 2003) and a 5-year follow-up (McIntosh, Carter, Bulik, Frampton, & Joyce, 2011).

Evidence for Cue Exposure as a Second-Stage Therapy

Other research indicates that cue exposure is beneficial in addressing binge eating in patients who do not respond to CBT (where that CBT does not involve cue exposure). In a study of six adult women with chronic binge-eating difficulties who did not respond to CBT, cue exposure was effective in eliminating binge-eating episodes and reducing other ED features. Those gains were well maintained at two separate follow-up time points over the next 3 years (Toro et al., 2003). In a larger study of over 20 adolescents with BN who did not benefit from CBT (Martinez-Mallén et al., 2007), exposure to binge cues yielded significantly reduced binge-eating frequency, as well as decreases in both self-reported and physiological measures of anxiety.

EVIDENCE FOR OTHER EXPOSURE STRATEGIES

Whereas the evidence considered in this chapter has predominantly focused on exposure addressing eating-related fears/avoidance, body image anxiety, and binge-eating cues, there is some research support for other forms of exposure in the treatment of EDs. For instance, some of the earliest research using exposure aimed to enhance tolerance of urges to vomit by exposing patients with BN to food consumption (e.g., specific types of food or quantities of food) that triggered the urge to vomit. Patients were then instructed to resist the urge to vomit and focus on the anxiety-provoking sensations and thoughts. Although a single case study provided support for this approach (Rosen & Leitenberg, 1982), a small follow-up controlled trial showed minimal benefit as compared to standard CBT (Leitenberg, Rosen, Gross, Nudelman, & Vara, 1988).

More recently, Levinson, Rapp, and Riley (2014) developed an imaginal exposure therapy intervention to assist ED patients in addressing their most feared concerns related to gaining weight. Although in its infancy, this intervention shows promising outcomes in decreasing eating-related anxiety and avoidance (Levinson et al., 2014). Additionally, several researchers have developed virtual reality paradigms involving exposure to computer-based simulations of ED-relevant stimuli, such as virtual grocery stores, restaurants, kitchens, clothing stores, and even a patient's own body size/shape (e.g., Gutiérrez-Maldonado, Ferrer-García, Caqueo-Urízar, & Moreno, 2010). A recent review found that virtual reality exposure appears to have a beneficial impact on an array of ED symptoms (Clus, Larsen, Lemey, & Berrouiguet, 2018).

SUMMARY

This chapter has given you an overview of the current available evidence supporting the use of exposure therapy for EDs. Although further research is needed because the existing research base is relatively small compared to very large exposure literature for anxiety disorders, exposure does appear to be an effective approach for addressing a range of key transdiagnostic features in EDs, including eating-related fear and avoidance, body image anxiety, compulsive body checking and avoidance, and binge-eating and purging behaviors. These results are found in a range of study types, from single case studies to large, methodically rigorous controlled trials. It is important to note that several of the studies reviewed in this chapter showed that exposure was helpful for patients who had been previously unable to derive benefit from viable alternative treatments. Therefore, you might find that exposure can offer a critical "missing element" in treatment protocols that have a reasonably strong evidence base and yet leave room for improvement in outcomes. You should also note that the therapeutic benefits of exposure treatments are well-maintained over time. In light of high rates of relapse in EDs (Keel et al., 2005), remember that a high dose of exposure has a good chance of helping to prevent your ED patients from relapsing. As previously noted, this evidence is less well developed in younger cases, although the development of ARFID as a diagnostic construct and the underpinning role of anxiety in many such cases makes it likely that such evidence will be forthcoming.

> **Summary Points—Part 1: Theoretical Basis of Exposure for Eating Disorders**
>
> - EDs have a number of common features across diagnoses, including avoidance and safety behaviors.
> - The use of those behaviors makes EDs a clear domain where exposure therapy can and should be used.
> - An understanding of the use of exposure therapy in anxiety disorders is valuable for understanding how to apply it in EDs.
> - Different ways of implementing exposure therapy are available, to be used as necessary in the individual case.
> - Exposure therapy is extremely effective for anxiety disorders.
> - We need to be able to explain the reasons why exposure therapy is indicated for EDs (overlap of content with anxiety disorders; the comorbidity of EDs and anxiety disorders; the inherent presence of exposure in therapies that work for EDs).
> - Explaining the value of exposure therapy for EDs depends on our understanding and communicating the theoretical basis and the evidence to support its use.
> - Knowing how to apply exposure is more important than knowing definitely how it works.
> - An inhibitory learning approach to exposure is likely to be particularly effective.
> - We have lots to learn from how planned exposure is delivered in anxiety disorders.
> - Different forms of exposure (particularly food-based, body-focused, and cue-based) are evidenced to be effective for EDs, and will be addressed in Part 3.

PART 2

Preparing to Start Exposure Therapy

6

Functional Assessment of Eating Disorders and Their Maintenance

As noted in Chapter 4, one parallel between EDs and anxiety-based disorders is the functional relationship between fears and the associated avoidance and safety behaviors. You will find that functional assessment is critical to your success as an exposure therapist. Understanding what your patient fears, as well as how he has typically coped using avoidant and safety behaviors, is necessary if you want to design useful exposure tasks. For instance, two patients may both report fearing weight gain, and they may engage in similar patterns of avoidance and use similar safety behaviors. Yet one patient may fear weight gain because weight gain is predicted to be uncontrollable and never ending, whereas the other patient may fear that only a moderate amount of weight gain will result in social repercussions that are viewed as intolerable (Murray et al., 2016; Waller & Mountford, 2015). As you learned in Chapter 3, a key component of successful exposure is that it violates the relevant harm expectancy, and your patients learn what they need to learn. Thus, you need to design exposure tasks so that they are most likely to violate the critical harm expectancy, which clearly differs across those two patients. If you do not understand what your patients fear or how your patients use avoidant and safety behaviors to manage their fears, you will not be able to do this successfully.

> Jessica, a 50-year-old mother of three teenage girls, reported an on-and-off history of dietary restriction and purging behaviors. Jessica restricted her eating throughout her teenage years and early 20s and noted that she was always very proud of how slender she kept her body. She also reported significant reinforcement for staying thin from family, friends, and dating partners. Following her marriage, based on Jessica's self-reported retrospective weight, she typically hovered around an 18 body mass index (BMI) until the birth of her first child. After this, Jessica found herself struggling to lose the "baby weight," particularly around her abdominal area. She reported that fatigue from staying up at night with her new baby reduced her ability to restrict her intake, and she began gaining weight. Jessica was terrified the

weight would continue to accumulate, and she would become "a whale," which would result in her husband leaving her for another woman. To reduce the chance of weight gain, she began to induce vomiting anytime she ate what she considered to be unacceptably large amounts of food given the circumstances. Later, Jessica began using coffee enemas after reading about them in an alternative health magazine article. Jessica stopped vomiting and using enemas during each of her subsequent two pregnancies but resumed once she gave birth to try to lose her pregnancy weight. At the time of assessment, Jessica's BMI was 19.7, and she described herself as "unacceptably fat and flabby." Jessica sought treatment after two of her daughters caught her vomiting after dinner. Jessica feared they would follow in her footsteps and develop EDs, which is why she sought treatment. Jessica noted she had tried to stop on her own but was unable. She reported being surprised she couldn't stop, because she "hated" vomiting and really wanted to set a good example for her daughters.

In the case of Jessica, you can clearly see that her ED behaviors are driven by several fears as well as some positive reinforcement. Jessica found maintaining a very thin body very reinforcing and experienced the loss of that body quite anxiety-provoking, secondary to a fear of uncontrollable weight gain. Jessica also feared that weight gain would have the social repercussion of losing her husband. Her vomiting and enema behaviors served the function of reducing her anxiety about weight gain.

FUNCTIONAL ASSESSMENT: OVERVIEW

Given the substantial medical morbidity associated with EDs, any functional assessment of EDs must include consideration of safety as a starting point. You will need to identify, monitor, and, where appropriate, respond to any physical and/or other risks (e.g., Birmingham & Treasure, 2010). In the case of Jessica, this included assessment of the frequency of her vomiting and use of enemas as well as periodic electrolyte testing. Jessica's clinician also provided her with psychoeducation about the potential risks associated with coffee enemas (Keum et al., 2010).

Once any risks are identified and managed, your next step is to fully understand how the ED "functions" so that you can plan treatment. CBT models of EDs are primarily focused on the maintenance of problems, considering origins only to the degree that they enhance your understanding and help you to reduce risk of relapse (e.g., Fairburn, Cooper & Shafran, 2003). This chapter will show you that many ED symptoms and related behaviors can function as avoidant or safety behaviors, both of which serve the function of reducing anxiety. This understanding will help you to more effectively conceptualize EDs from an anxiety perspective. In other words, by the end of this chapter, you should be able to connect what you learned in Part 1 of this book even more clearly to your ED patients and their behaviors. When you embark on treatment, you will carefully consider ED behaviors both in your initial assessment and beyond, identifying those that serve as avoidant or safety behaviors. These behaviors typically can be most successfully addressed using exposure therapy.

Your aim is to understand ED behaviors from a functional perspective. That perspective recognizes that behaviors and symptoms that appear to be pathological in the longer term are maintained because they provide a functional (or useful) outcome in the shorter term. Frequently this function is to reduce anxiety. So, behaviors that might seem irrational in isolation (e.g., the patient who vomits and says that they hate doing so) actually make sense when you understand that the behaviors have a positive short-term function (e.g., reducing postbinge fear of weight gain). However, ED behaviors also may serve other functions as well, and you will need to understand those functions for each of your patients. For example, while patients often report that they dislike bingeing, that behavior can have the immediate positive function of reducing a range of negative emotions other than anxiety (e.g., shame), and it also reduces hunger in patients who are otherwise restricting their intake. Jessica reported being surprised that she couldn't stop vomiting on her own despite hating it. Careful functional assessment, however, revealed that in addition to reducing anxiety related to weight gain, vomiting and using enemas also produced the positively reinforcing feeling of being "empty." Thus, vomiting and enema use

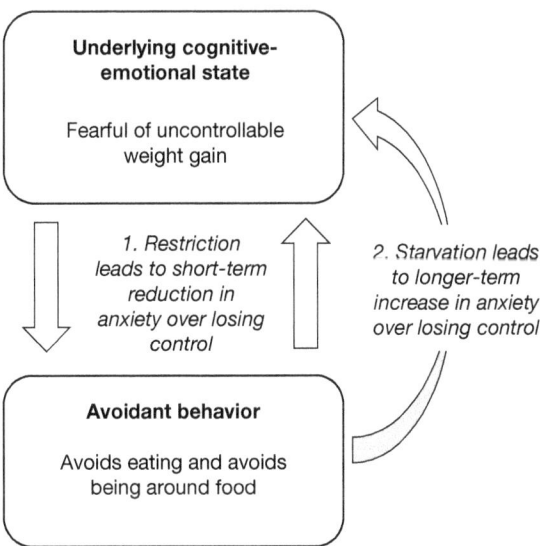

Figure 6.1. A simple avoidant/safety behavior, where restriction has the short-term positive effect of reducing fear of uncontrollable weight gain (1), but has the longer-term consequence of starvation, raising anxiety about such weight gain (2).

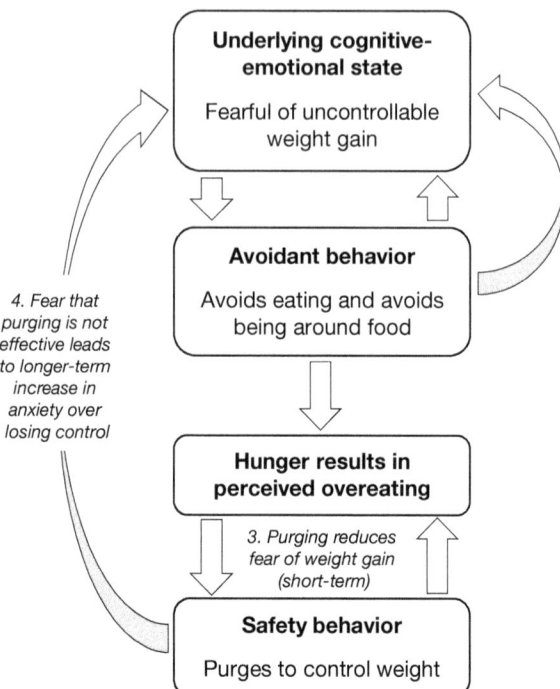

Figure 6.2. A short chain of avoidant/safety behaviors. Restriction (Figure 6.1) enhances hunger and triggers eating, resulting using the safety behavior of purging to reduce the effects of eating (3) in Figure 6.2. However, concern about whether the purging will work results in longer term enhancement of fears about uncontrollable weight gain (4) in Figure 6.2.

were both positively (made Jessica feel empty) and negatively (reduced anxiety) reinforced in the short term. Figure 6.1 provides an example of how one common ED avoidant behavior can function, demonstrating both the positive benefits in the short term as well the negative long-term outcomes. Figure 6.2 shows how a number of such behaviors can chain together to enhance the maintenance of multiple ED symptoms.

It is important to remember that the pattern of avoidant/safety behaviors that you will need to address can change over the course of therapy. For instance, in the case of Jessica, her clinician initially targeted eating and purging behaviors. Later, he targeted behaviors that contributed to ongoing poor body image (e.g., body avoidance, body comparison). However, keep in mind that most avoidant/safety behaviors will have been part of your patient's repertoire for many years. Therefore, if such behaviors are seen at the initial assessment, you will likely need to directly target them at some point during the course of therapy.

IDENTIFYING THE SPECIFIC FUNCTIONAL ROLE(S) OF AVOIDANCE AND SAFETY BEHAVIORS IN EATING DISORDERS: WHAT TO ASK AT ASSESSMENT (AND BEYOND)?

A comprehensive assessment of an ED should cover a range of domains (see Waller et al., 2007, for additional detail). These will include the following.

- Eating patterns (e.g., restriction, overeating and binge eating)
- Eating safety behaviors (e.g., eating very slowly or quickly, eating in very small bits, removing oil using napkins; see Chapter 4 for more discussion)
- Purging and other compensatory behaviors
- Avoidance of feared information (e.g., not wanting to be weighed or to know their weight)
- Specific fears (e.g., being unable engage in physical activity, weight gain, shopping)
- Patterns of social interaction relating to eating and body image (e.g., mind-reading, reassurance seeking, avoidance of social eating) and body-related behaviors (e.g., avoidance of seeing one's body; wearing very loose clothes, checking one's body; comparison with others).

Each of these can be conceptualized as a behavior that has both short-term positive benefits and long-term negative outcomes, as detailed in Table 4.1.

You should consider any such avoidant/safety behaviors at the initial assessment and monitor for any changes as therapy progresses. Remember that not all behaviors will be evident at the start of therapy, in part because some behaviors become so habitual, your patients lose awareness of them. Methods of assessment include the following:

1. *Questions asked routinely at interview.* Such questions are relatively natural to ask in an ED assessment (e.g., "Do you use mirrors at home?"; "Tell me about your normal pattern of eating. Let's start with what you had to eat across the course of yesterday?"; "How do you feel emotionally just before and just after you binge?"). Both avoidant and safety behaviors often come up in the course of the initial interview even when not addressed directly, and you should be alert to the possibility that you can gather a lot of key functional assessment information in this way.
2. *Directly asking your patient about specific feared objects and situations.* These fears are likely to become evident during the routine interview. Fears might include specific foods, clothing items, activities, body posture/positions, periods of physical inactivity during long car trips, etc.

3. *Asking friends, family, carers, and other professionals about the behaviors used.* This is one method for eliciting information about behaviors that your patients may no longer be aware of using, or the effects of those behaviors. For instance, you can ask about how much your patients seek reassurance or compare themselves with others. Asking such questions also can assist in helping others to see how they might be contributing to the problem, and how they might be able to help your patient to change (see Chapter 17). Gaining awareness of such symptom "accommodation" is an important step toward engaging others in helping your patients to engage in exposure-based methods (e.g., normative eating) within FBT, CBT, and other approaches.

Jessica's husband, Carl, had long been aware of his wife's ED but had backed off from asking her to change. After talking with Jessica's clinician, Carl realized how his own avoidance behaviors played a role in maintaining her ED. More specifically, Carl had stopped asking Jessica to eat more (even when she felt lightheaded and had to hold on to furniture for balance) because he didn't want to upset her. Jessica claimed fighting made it harder to eat, so Carl tried his best to keep their interactions "light." He reported hoping she would eat simply because they were not fighting about her eating behavior. He similarly ignored her purging behaviors and turned on the television so their daughters wouldn't inadvertently hear their mother vomiting.

---

4. *Established measures of avoidance and safety behaviors* (e.g., food diaries; questionnaires regarding body checking and comparison). Carefully consider your options when selecting which measures you want to use with a given patient. Remember that you can personalize any pack of psychometric measures that you send home with your patient to be completed. So while you might routinely include a questionnaire that you would use monitor eating pathology (e.g., the Eating Disorders Examination-Questionnaire; Fairburn & Beglin, 2008), you might also add a measure of body image avoidance (e.g., Body Image Avoidance Questionnaire; Rosen, Srebnik, Saltzberg, & Wendt, 1991) or body checking (e.g., Body Checking Questionnaire; Reas, Whisenhunt, Netemeyer, & Williamson, 2002). This personalization is likely to enhance your patient's engagement and completion of the measures.
5. *Observation in the session.* Observing your patient's behavior in session is a key therapy skill. Early observation of how your patient acts in the session can help you to identify material to work on to develop effective therapy. Sample patient behaviors that you should look out for include patients being reluctant to be weighed or to know their weight (see Chapter 12 for further discussion); patients comparing themselves with

others in the waiting area or with you directly; patients wearing baggy or very heavy clothing; and patients engaging in body-checking behaviors.

Having identified the core avoidant/safety behaviors that are commonly used by your patient and the function that each serves, it is critical to explain the common theme to your patient (short-term benefit vs. longer term negative effects). Then you need to explain that there is a method for addressing each of those behaviors so that your patient can learn two key lessons:

1. The feared short-term outcome typically does not happen when your patient does not use the avoidant/safety behavior (e.g., not using extreme restriction does not have to result in uncontrollable weight gain). Further, if a perceived negative outcome does happen, it will be more tolerable than expected (e.g., any weight gain is likely to be minimal and short-lived or controllable if weight gain is necessary).
2. Using the avoidant/safety behavior makes the feared outcomes more likely (e.g., restriction makes binge eating more likely, resulting in the feared weight gain that your patient was trying to avoid in the first place).

Those two lessons are addressed explicitly in Chapter 7, which provides more detail as to how to educate your patient to the rationale for and the value of exposure therapy.

SUMMARY

Your patients are individuals, who will experience different symptoms. Your task is to understand those symptoms and plan treatment accordingly. That understanding is much easier if you focus your assessment on the short- and long-term functions that the ED behaviors serve. Identifying those functions will allow you to engage your patient and their family in making changes, as they understand that their existing responses are not working and are worsening the ED symptoms.

7
Explaining Exposure Therapy to Your Patients

As discussed in Chapter 4, it is critical that you understand the rationale for using exposure with your ED patients so that you can use the relevant techniques appropriately. Later in this book (Chapters 18 and 19), we discuss the reasons why so many clinicians often fail to deliver exposure therapy appropriately. These reasons are important for all of us to consider, because few clinicians are completely immune to the urge to back off from exposure. Indeed, exposure is often anxiety-provoking for the clinician—not just the patient! Moreover, if you supervise other clinicians, you will need to be on the lookout for the problems discussed in those chapters.

In this chapter, however, we will assume that you are well educated in the rationale for exposure and are committed to delivering it as accurately as possible, without "skipping" what are often perceived as uncomfortable elements. Your first task in embarking on exposure is to educate your patients about the problematic avoidance and safety behaviors that they use and then providing a compelling rationale for the use of exposure therapy. The rationale for using exposure therapy needs to be personalized enough for your patients to understand how it applies to them and should also include a discussion of the basic principles. In the following discussion, we focus on strategies you can use to explain exposure therapy to your ED patients to engage them in the necessary elements of their treatment.

Let us start by considering a case for which it will be important to think through why we need to explain exposure, when we should do so, and how we can explain it effectively. In Clara's case, it is important to understand her ED history, her treatment history, and why this is the first time that she has been introduced to exposure therapy as a method:

> Clara is a 20-year-old university student, with a 6-year history of dietary restriction and vomiting. She began restricting her eating after being teased in school for being chubby. Later she learned about vomiting while watching a documentary on eating disorders. Clara lost a significant amount of weight

and was widely praised by both peers and others. When she reached a body mass index of 17, her parents took her to her pediatrician out of fear of the continuing weight loss. Clara was then referred to a dietitian but made little progress. She eventually terminated with the dietitian because she was tired of being "nagged" about her eating. To appease her parents, she started seeing a clinician whose approach focused on uncovering the underlying reason for Clara's ED. Clara liked the clinician and also liked the fact that she didn't have to focus on her eating behaviors in therapy. Ten months ago, however, Clara started binge eating in secret, and her weight began climbing. Clara decided to seek out treatment with a new clinician to put an end to the binge eating and gain control over her eating.

WHY DO WE NEED TO EXPLAIN EXPOSURE THERAPY TO OUR PATIENTS?

Psychoeducation regarding the rationale for exposure therapy is a critical component of exposure, for one simple reason: patients who do not understand why they are doing something, particularly a very hard and aversive something, are unlikely to actively participate in exposure (and thus benefit from it). When you present the rationale for exposure therapy, you are selling both the technique and the logic behind the technique to your patients. Your success in doing so plays a critical role in the success of exposure.

This argument is illustrated, in part, by Cowdrey's (2014) work, which examined ED patients' perceptions of the helpfulness of different techniques that they should have experienced in CBT. Three exposure-based methods were considered—weighing, dietary change, and introducing feared situations and foods. The patients were divided into three groups: those for whom the technique had never been used during their course of CBT; those who had experienced the treatment method but who had no memory of the clinician having explained the rationale; and those who had experienced both the technique and the clinician explanation of the rationale. For each technique, the patients who had received both the explanation and the technique reported gaining the most benefit.

To summarize, ED patients like Clara are more likely to find exposure-based methods helpful if we explain the reason for using them. Doing so will also have the effect of increasing your patients' expectations for treatment success, which will assist in motivating your patients to follow through with the actual treatment. Doing so also typically has the positive side effect of improving the therapeutic relationship because you demonstrate to your patients that you view their behaviors as both understandable and treatable.

As will be seen later in the book (Chapter 19), not all clinicians are happy to use exposure-based methods. Cowdrey (2014), however, has identified another group of clinicians who use those techniques without providing sufficient rationale. To maximize patient engagement and benefit with someone like Clara, you need to both explain the technique and use it correctly.

WHEN SHOULD WE EXPLAIN EXPOSURE THERAPY TO OUR PATIENTS?

As we discussed in Part 1, exposure therapy is a core component of CBT for EDs. It also is often an implicit element of other therapies (e.g., the family meal in FBT and weighing patients openly in a range of evidence-based therapies). In CBT, as with most evidence-based therapies for EDs, elements of exposure emerge very early in treatment (e.g., change in diet; trying feared foods; weighing your patient). Therefore, you will want to provide the rationale for exposure to your patients at the beginning of therapy. This early explanation can be particularly engaging with a patient like Clara, as you can use it to incorporate thoughts about why her previous work with other clinicians (which did not include exposure) was not effective. You engender hope when you can explain why previous treatment results do not need to predict future results.

You also will find it useful to reiterate the key points of exposure when moving to addressing new symptoms. For example, evidence-based CBT includes substantial use of exposure starting with the first session, during which you introduce dietary changes. However, exposure also is used to address emotionally driven behaviors and body image anxiety and avoidance later in therapy. Our experience has been that some clinicians assume that explaining exposure once is adequate. Yet, the presenting features are different at each of these stages, and you cannot assume that your patients will be able to apply early explanations of exposure aimed at one set of symptoms to other situations and symptoms.

There is a caveat to the recommendation to introduce exposure right at the start of treatment. Remember that exposure is *most likely* to be successful when your patients *voluntarily* engage in exposure, because a patient who undergoes exposure involuntarily typically will find a way to engage in covert (i.e., hidden) avoidant and safety behaviors. These can markedly reduce the success of exposure. This is important to remember given that early "exposure" for severely underweight AN patients in inpatient treatment may not be voluntary (where the primary concern is restoring weight, stabilizing medical concerns, and improving nutrition). In this case, patients may not learn what they need to learn during what appears to be exposure therapy, secondary to covert avoidance and safety behaviors, or because early weight restoration actually initially confirms their worst fears (i.e., the harm expectancy of significant weight gain actually happens; Murray et al., 2016). Thus, it may be prudent in some cases to hold off introducing exposure to extremely malnourished patients with AN in inpatient treatment until engaging in treatment becomes somewhat more voluntary. This requires team decisions about when the focus needs to be biological safety versus engagement of the patient as an active participant in exposure therapy, and communicating with your patients and their families about the need to transition to the use of exposure-based methods.

However, there is also some evidence that, in some cases, malnourished patients with AN *can* in fact derive good therapeutic benefit from introducing exposure early in the course of treatment as long as they receive a solid rationale for exposure (Farrell, Bowie, et al., 2019). The lesson here is that an effective rationale is crucial in ensuring that your patients are volitionally engaging in exposure versus perceiving themselves as "forced" to comply with unreasonable demands.

In summary, you typically will want to introduce the rationale for exposure to a patient like Clara at the beginning of therapy. At this point in treatment, exposure largely will be focused on changes in eating. You should then be prepared to explain how the same principles apply when moving on to other symptoms. Particularly if later symptoms do not respond to exposure therapy, you should consider whether you need to revisit the rationale for exposure, making the connection to the specific symptom that is under consideration.

HOW SHOULD WE EXPLAIN EXPOSURE THERAPY TO OUR PATIENTS?

First, it is important to remember that the core elements of exposure are relatively easy to explain—your patient needs to fully experience anxiety (exposure) without use of avoidance or a safety behavior (response prevention). That way, she can learn safety and discover that she can tolerate anxiety better than expected. *Safety learning* typically means learning that a feared outcome does not come to pass (i.e., the harm expectancy is clearly violated). However, it also may mean learning that a feared outcome was simply not as intolerable as predicted. In this case, the harm expectancy would be that the feared outcome was intolerable.

Few patients struggle to understand the basic principles of exposure, even though they can find it scary to implement it. To overcome the natural reluctance to engage in exposure that most of your patients (like Clara) will experience, begin by explaining how exposure works. Depending on your therapeutic style and what is effective for a given patient, consider using clinical examples, analogies, and historical review, as well as connections to what your patient has previously done (or not done) in therapy.

Explaining the Process and Mechanisms of Exposure

We typically start by explaining to patients that their symptoms are entirely understandable, because they have served a function for so long. Your aim is to avoid any sense you are blaming your patients, and this includes not joining in their self-blame. Therefore, we use an approach that is similar to Linehan's (1993) comprehensive validation: we stress that we understand our patient's use of the behavior, given the context where it developed and the lack of opportunity to change to date. However, we also stress that we do not believe that our patient has to be stuck with their behaviors, beliefs, and emotions. The following is a typical explanation of how avoidance and safety behaviors work. Note that although the literature distinguishes between *avoidance* (i.e., stimuli or situations avoided to reduce anxiety) and *safety behaviors* (acts designed to neutralize anxiety when avoidance is not possible), we do not find that distinction is useful for patients. As such, in the following dialogue, Clara's clinician lumps avoidance behaviors and safety behaviors under one term—safety behaviors.

> **Clinician:** So, if I have it right, you have been restricting your food intake (*avoidance behavior*) and using vomiting (*safety behavior*) for about 6 years, since you were 14. You started out trying to lose weight, but now you use them in an attempt to keep your weight from going up. Even though it isn't working and your weight is going up slowly, you keep trying both behaviors because you are worried that your weight will shoot up uncontrollably if you don't use them. Is that right?
> **Clara:** Yes, that's it. I thought I had found a great way to be slim; then I thought I could at least keep my weight stable. Now, I just keep failing to keep my weight from going up, but I am terrified that I will get fatter and fatter if I stop trying.
> **Clinician:** That makes sense. I can see how you developed those patterns in how you coped. I am sure that there were lots of reasons why you might have wanted to be slim in the first place. However, I am going to focus more on what is keeping your eating disorder symptoms going now—what we call "maintenance." I need to introduce you to a way of making sense of what you have been doing, so that we can help you to get out of that pattern.
> **Clara:** Okay. I am not really sure what I am doing makes any sense though.
> **Clinician:** Well, let's see. The first thing that I want you to learn about is what we call "safety behaviors." A safety behavior is what happens when you do something that works in the short term by making you less anxious, but makes things worse in the longer term. So you start by restricting, because that makes you less worried about gaining weight, but that then makes you hungry, and you start worrying even more about breaking your rules and overeating so you try even harder to stick to your diet. So dieting is your first safety behavior, because it makes you feel better at first, but ends up making you more worried. Does that make sense?
> **Clara:** That makes sense to me, yes.
> **Clinician:** However, your body takes over, and you end up eating something that is on your "forbidden foods" list—sometimes in quite large amounts. That makes you panic, and the only way that you can stop that extra anxiety is to get rid of the food by making yourself sick, in the hope that vomiting will get rid of all the food. Initially, vomiting reduces your anxiety, but over time, the fact that you vomit makes you feel even worse

>about yourself and adds to the pressure on your body to eat more. So you end up feeling much worse about yourself and far more out of control. That vomiting is your second safety behavior. Again does that make sense to you?
>
>**Clara:** Yes. I see what you mean.
>
>**Clinician:** Is it a surprise to you, or does it fit with what you already knew about yourself?
>
>**Clara:** Well, I sort of knew it, but didn't want it to be that way. I sort of hoped that every time I starved myself or threw up, that would be it, and it would work so that I didn't have to worry any more. Instead, my weight has just kept creeping up, and I hate that.
>
>**Clinician:** That is often the way with safety behaviors—you keep doing them even when your rational side says to stop. But now it is time to deal with that anxiety in a more productive way and to learn that your weight likely doesn't have to go up and up like that anymore.

It is important to note that this discussion with Clara was directed toward making the argument as compelling as possible, so that she is ready to move on to seeing the logic behind the use of exposure (as addressed in the following discussion). For example, the clinical summary was based as closely as possible on Clara's own experiences, and the clinician opened up the possibility that Clara "sort of knew" all this already. The aim is to persuade your patient to accept that their existing avoidant/safety behaviors might be working in the short term (reducing immediate anxiety), but that they are failing to work in the long term, often worsening the feelings and outcomes that your patient is trying to avoid.

Having explained safety behaviors, Clara's clinician next explains how exposure works, with the aim of ensuring that Clara sees the logic of giving this approach a try.

>**Clinician:** Now, you have a choice about whether you want to change or not. I know that you have tried therapies before that were largely about *talking* about how you wanted to be different. However, all the evidence says that the best way of getting out of the safety behavior trap is to *do* things differently.
>
>**Clara:** But what does that look like?
>
>**Clinician:** The main aim is to help you learn some things you need to learn. First, you learn that if you don't use your safety behaviors, you will feel anxious for a short while. However, you will also learn several useful lessons. First, you will learn that you are tougher than you think, and you can tolerate more anxiety than you expect. Basically, you learn that you don't need to avoid your anxiety because you can handle it. Equally important, you also will learn that your worst fears either don't come true or are not as bad as you thought they would be—we call this safety learning. The great thing about learning anxiety tolerance and safety learning is

that you don't have the downside of the negative long-term consequences of using the safety behaviors. So, if you don't restrict when you have the urge, you feel worried in the short term, but you don't have the long-term worry about losing control or the need to make yourself sick. Likewise, if you don't vomit when you get the urge to, you might worry for a while about the effects of what you just ate, but long term you don't have the physical pressures to eat even more and the slow weight gain.

Clara: So how do I know that will work for me? What if it all goes wrong?

Clinician: Well, I can give you a handout based on some research that should help you [see the appendix for handout]. It shows how everyone worries when they first try changing their eating but how that gets easier after a few sessions, and you will start seeing the positives. However, the only way that you can be sure that it will work for you is if you try it yourself.

Clara: Okay. So if I wanted to find out if it works for me, what would I have to do?

Clinician: This is where we use a technique called "exposure therapy." The first part is where we ask you to confront the things that cause the anxiety—say, eating foods that scare you. Second, we ask you to allow the anxiety to be present without trying to escape it and learn that your worst fears don't come to pass or are more tolerable than you anticipate. That means not using any safety behaviors, like vomiting or exercising. We call that "response prevention." So there are two parts: exposure to the thing that scares you and not using your safety behaviors.

Clara: And the idea is that I learn that eating the food is something I can handle?

Clinician: That is part of it, but it is also important that you learn that your safety behavior is a bad thing for you, as it makes you more anxious in the long term and keeps your eating disorder going. Does that make sense to you?

Clara: Well, it sounds scary, because you are asking me to put up with changing how I eat and how I cope with my fear. But I think I see how it could be good for me to change. And it would be good to see the handout about it working for other people.

Clinician: Thinking further ahead in your treatment, we will also look at using this "exposure with response prevention" approach for other symptoms. Based on what we talked about in your assessment, if you can learn how to address your anxiety this way now, it will be useful when we are looking at your body image issues later on.

Clara: Oh, that would be so good—though I bet that will be scary too.

Clinician: Scary in the short term, but helpful for how you feel about your body for years to come.

In this example, Clara's clinician has outlined the principles of exposure with response prevention (i.e., exposure therapy), linking them to Clara's own anxiety and avoidant/safety behaviors. The clinician also has checked that this makes sense to Clara and allowed her the opportunity to *explain* her understanding of the rationale versus simply acknowledging her understanding. The importance of behavioral change ("doing" therapies) has been stressed, compared with therapies that are "talk-based." Clara's clinician has also stressed that the positive longer-term impact of exposure therapy and response prevention is common in EDs (Waller, Evans, & Pugh, 2013), even if Clara has never experienced it personally. Finally, the clinician linked the current use of exposure (for overcoming fears about changing eating patterns) with what Clara is likely to need later in her ED treatment. All of these elements will to be useful in engaging Clara in undertaking exposure therapy on an ongoing basis. This is important because your patients will not decide to engage in exposure once. They will have to make that decision repeatedly throughout therapy and repeatedly talk themselves into approaching aversive and fear-producing situations.

Use of Analogies to Explain the Impact of Exposure Therapy for Eating Disorders

When a patient finds it hard to understand the principles of exposure therapy, we often find that using simple analogies drawn from patients' past experiences is an effective method for communicating the key points.

> **Clinician:** Remember how you told me that you stayed with your ex for a long time, even though they were aggressive to you? That can happen when your safety behavior is to stay with what you know rather than risking change. It can feel safer to stick with the uncomfortable current situation, rather than face going through major changes where you do not know for certain what the outcome will be. So your safety behavior is to stay where you are. The short-term benefit is not having to do something scary where you cannot be sure about the outcome, but in long term things just get worse and worse.
>
> **Clara:** I get that. Staying where I am is not risky but it is unpleasant, and I will be more and more unhappy at the time—like I did when I was trying to patch up that relationship but couldn't make it work. If I had changed earlier and got out of that relationship, that would have been much better for me. I guess that means that I might be better off changing my eating sooner rather than later, rather than keep going with my safety behavior . . .
>
> **Clinician:** That's right – you just described exposure therapy.

Sometimes, this use of analogies can be made more effective by asking the patient to consider how they would explain exposure to someone else or how they would use it to overcome a relatively common problem. For example:

Clinician: So let's imagine that you have a friend who has been talking about wanting to learn to swim, so that they can swim with their children. However, they are worried about getting in the water and possibly drowning. Every time they go to the swimming pool, they dip in their toe in the water, and then run off. What would you advise them to do to be able to swim with their children?
Clara: That's pretty obvious—they just have to face up to it and get in the pool. If they keep running away, like a safety behavior, they are never going to achieve what they want to. I would tell them that it might be scary when they first get in, but they will soon learn that they don't drown, and then they can get to swim with the children.
Clinician: That makes sense. So what would you tell yourself about your own fears of starting to eat normally?
Clara: Well, it's the same thing, I suppose. I need to dive in and just do it.

In such cases, we routinely find that our patients can solve the problem for someone else with ease. Your job is to ensure that your patients see that this approach and solution apply to themselves, too.

Historical Review of Unintended Exposure Experiences

It can also be helpful to remind patients that they have almost certainly already "done" exposure in other domains in their life without realizing it, most commonly using exposure to overcome natural fears in childhood (e.g., riding tall rollercoasters, pedaling a bicycle without training wheels, jumping into the "deep end" of the swimming pool, etc.). Such reminders serve two important functions. First, they provide an opportunity to illustrate key aspects of the treatment rationale, such as expectancy violation and developing improved tolerance of fear. Second, they can help to increase patients' confidence in the treatment if they believe they are doing something that is not completely new to them.

Comparison With Other Disorders to Explain the Impact of Exposure Therapy for Eating Disorders

It is also possible to explain exposure therapy in terms of how one would address another disorder (that your patient is not experiencing). This comparison allows the patient to see what is needed more objectively.

Clinician: Imagine you had a friend who suffered from panic attacks, and every time they felt anxious they were afraid that they would have a heart attack. That would mean that whenever they felt the early signs of anxiety, then they would be likely to run away from the situation that they were in. That running away is their safety behavior, and it means that they start to believe that it is the running away that saves them from dying. However, the safety behavior means that they never get to learn that they would not really have a heart attack, and that they can tolerate their anxiety. So what do you think we should aim to do in that situation?

Clara: I suppose that it's clear enough. The safety behavior is running away to reduce the anxiety, so we would need to keep them there to face the anxiety and learn. That would be response prevention, wouldn't it?

Comparison with Previous Therapies

Many of our patients have had one or more previous experiences of therapy for their ED. As mentioned earlier, it can be valuable to discuss previous therapies with your patient to understand whether that therapy included an exposure element and whether that exposure was appropriately explained and implemented. We very often find that patients report that previous clinicians have not used or mentioned exposure for their ED, even when that therapy was described as CBT. This clinical impression is well supported by the literature on CBT for EDs (Cowdrey & Waller, 2015; Mulkens, de Vos, de Graff, & Walker, 2018; Waller, Stringer, & Meyer, 2012). Many patients describe that there was no pressure in therapy to change their eating, or that techniques were applied inadequately (e.g., the patient was weighed, but not told what their weight was).

When it is clear that your patient's previous therapies have not included adequate (or any) use of exposure therapy, that deficit should be highlighted as a surprising omission. For example:

Clinician: Well, I am not that surprised that you might feel a bit pessimistic about having CBT again, but I am worried that the problem is not that you didn't do well with CBT, but that you didn't really have CBT at all. All the books are very clear about what needs to happen in evidence-based CBT, and that didn't happen for you.

The aim is to help your patient to overcome any sense of being responsible for the previous therapy not working. In other words, you want your patients to attribute the failure of therapy externally, rather than internally. As clinicians, we also need to avoid terms like "treatment failure" or "resistant to treatment" when the therapy was inadequate or poorly delivered. You need to engender optimism about the therapy in your patients, and you want to maintain your own therapeutic optimism. That way, when you start developing your plans for exposure

Psychoeducation as Exposure

You should keep in mind that for some patients, psychoeducation, including but not limited to psychoeducation about exposure, has the potential to significantly raise their anxiety. Highly avoidant patients may want to avoid even talking about their fears and/or behaviors they find shameful. They also may want to avoid talking about facing their fears or stopping specific behaviors. This anxiety matters for several reasons.

1. Psychoeducation can provide your patients with the opportunity to learn that they can tolerate the anxiety they experience when talking about key topics (e.g., discussing exposure or the degree to which laxative use is relatively ineffective as a means of weight loss).
2. Psychoeducation provides an opportunity for you to demonstrate that you, as a clinician, will not back away from something just because it elicits anxiety. Indeed, if you are covering psychoeducation about exposure, you can use this as a concrete example in your discussion of exposure.
3. Their anxiety might reflect a reasonable response to real risk, which can be reduced by removing the threat. For instance, learning about the risk of physical harm from laxative abuse creates significant anxiety for some patients. In this case, their desire to avoid the anxiety-provoking stimulus (ongoing use of laxatives) can be useful. Fear and avoidance of things that realistically have a significant chance of real lasting harm is not pathological but reasonable and adaptive.
4. While you might fear that teaching your patient explicitly about the negative side of their ED will distress them and encourage them to leave therapy, the evidence suggests that the opposite is true. Fursland, Erceg-Hurn, Byrne, and McEvoy (2018) have shown that a single, relatively "robust" pretreatment psychoeducation session is associated with symptom reduction and greater progress of patients into treatment. In other words, exposure to information is not a negative experience, as it has positive consequences for the patient.

SUMMARY

Providing a rationale for exposure therapy to your patients is a key element to successful exposure, especially when it has not been used previously or has been used inadequately. Patients who do not understand what is involved are less likely to commit to what could seem like a scary departure from their normal patterns of avoidance and safety behaviors. Unless there is a clear reason not to do so, explain exposure to eating and food at the beginning of therapy but be prepared to come back to it later in treatment when using exposure for other targets (e.g., emotions, body image). The explanation itself can include direct education, analogies, historical review, and comparison with other disorders. Even psychoeducation itself can have an exposure element.

8
Planning Exposure Therapy With Your Patients

Having explained the principles of exposure therapy to your patient (Chapter 7), you now need to plan how and when you are going to ensure that it happens. Many clinicians and patients assume exposure will primarily take place in the clinician's office. However, given what we have already outlined in Chapter 3 about the theory underpinning exposure, it is important to stress that you will need to implement exposure in varied settings for it to be maximally effective. That way, your patients will have an opportunity to generalize their learning and understand that they are safe and can tolerate their anxiety in a wide range of situations. Such generalizability and intensity of learning reduces the likelihood of relapse and increases the probability that your patients will understand how to do exposure on their own if anxiety spontaneously returns.

ECOLOGICAL VALIDITY OF EXPOSURE THERAPY

Exposure will be most effective for your patients when it is ecologically valid—that is, related to their everyday life, in all its diversity. Therefore, when planning exposure to overcome your patient's anxiety and change avoidant/safety behaviors (e.g., restriction, body checking, purging, etc.), you will need to consider your patients' concerns within the broad spectrum of their lives. For example, Chloe exercised excessively after every (small) meal in an effort to reduce her anxiety. This behavior could not be addressed adequately in the clinic, so Chloe's clinician worked with her to engage in exposure in everyday situations:

Clinician: So you are exercising several times a day, after you eat any meal, however small that might be. Is that right?
Chloe: That's right. If I didn't, I am scared that my weight would just fly up because of all the food that I have eaten.
Clinician: To help me understand, when is the last time that this happened, what had you eaten, and what exercise did you do?

Chloe: That was this morning. I had eaten a bagel with cream cheese, because you said that I should have some carbs for breakfast. I was okay with the bagel—I have been having them for two weeks now, without any weight gain. But I started to panic that the cream cheese might not really have been low-fat, so I decided to have a run to burn off the calories. I ran along the river for about an hour before going to work.

Clinician: And did that work for you? Did you feel better or see any change in your weight?

Chloe: Well, I checked. My weight didn't change, and I felt much calmer after the run. But then I started to feel hungry again and worried about overeating again. So I haven't had lunch yet, in case I binge.

Clinician: So the running calmed you down initially, but not for long, because your body started fighting back and wanting more fuel? That was what you got out of all that work?

Chloe: It doesn't make sense, now that we talk about it like that, but I was really anxious after that bagel, and going for a run was the only thing that I could think of that might calm me down.

Clinician: So you said you panicked because the cream cheese might not have really been low fat. What were you afraid was going to happen as a result?

Chloe: That I would blow up like a balloon.

Clinician: Can you be more precise than that? How much weight did you think you would put on?

Chloe: Well, any amount of weight is awful, but I was so anxious I was sure I was going to see two or more extra kilos on the scale.

Clinician: Okay. Remember when we talked about exposure therapy? What do you think I am likely to say to the idea that the run was the only thing that that you could do to cope?

Chloe: I suppose that it is about running being a safety behavior and that if I had held off from running, I would have learned that I could tolerate my anxiety.

Clinician: Great. What else might you have learned?

Chloe: I guess that a regular amount of cream cheese wouldn't make me gain a ton of weight.

Clinician: That is a pretty good analysis, but it goes a bit further. Your safety behavior of running used up quite a bit of energy, leaving you hungry and scared that you might binge. So, like all safety behaviors, not only do you not learn that you can tolerate your anxiety better than you think and that the feared outcome isn't as bad or as likely as you think, your safety behavior actually increases the risk of the very thing that you were scared of in the first place—overeating, in this case. So, what would be a good alternative?

Chloe: I suppose it is the obvious. When I get the urge to go for a run because I am anxious, I should delay and accept my anxiety.

Clinician: Right. So let me ask a question: If you hadn't been anxious about gaining weight, what would you have done during that time?

Chloe: Well, my plan had been to call my sister.

Clinician: So why didn't you call her?

Chloe: Because I ran instead . . .

Clinician: So is it safe to say that you believed that just doing what you would ordinarily do with that time was going to lead you to blow up like a balloon after eating a bagel and cream cheese?

Chloe: I guess so. Talking to my sister doesn't burn a lot of calories. I don't have good mobile service so I can't even pace a lot when talking to her. I pretty much need to sit in this one chair if I don't want her cutting in and out.

Clinician: So part of what you may need to learn is what?

Chloe: That I can eat and then do something sedentary, feel anxious, but in the end, be okay . . .

Clinician: I think so . . .

Chloe: What if I want to go for a run anyway sometime later because I actually like running along the river, can I?

Clinician: Absolutely. It is fine to exercise for positive reasons, like feeling fitter or just plain enjoying it. Just not immediately to block out the anxiety or burn calories or because you feel you "have to." So how could you make sure that you learn that exercise can be for fun, rather than to cope with what you have eaten?

Chloe: Well, it is like I said, when I get that urge to exercise after eating, I need to do something sedentary and deal with my anxiety. Then I can learn to eat like a normal person. And, I can exercise when I want to, rather than feeling compelled to.

You will notice that none of this exposure work (not exercising when Chloe feels anxious after eating a normal, although small, meal as part of her everyday life) could be carried out realistically in the clinic, in a way that had any ecological validity. While her clinician could get her to eat and then not exercise for 45 minutes in a therapy session, that would be a very constrained piece of learning, and Chloe is unlikely to learn what she needs to learn out in her daily life.

It is critical that Chloe identify these types of patterns when they arise (e.g., using a diary to note when the urge to exercise comes along and how it is linked to her eating). She then needs to have an exposure plan regarding how to prevent her safety behavior and accept the ensuing anxiety (e.g., a flashcard with sedentary alternatives to her safety behavior of running to burn calories). Rather than just conducting exposure in the clinic for this sort of situation, our job is to prepare Chloe for doing this work in the real world on a regular basis. Therefore, you need to prepare the diaries and flashcards with your patients, so that they can put their understanding into operation at the appropriate times. Remember that many patients need these aids to guide them precisely because they are so anxious. While it might be the case that some patients (e.g., younger clients) need more support (e.g., parent coaching), you should be careful to use those to ensure that exposure is delivered appropriately, rather than contributing to reducing the anxiety in the form of avoidance or a safety behavior.

TWO LEARNING OPPORTUNITIES

Your goal in getting your patients to undertake these behaviors in their everyday lives is really twofold. First, obviously, you want your patients to learn that they can tolerate their anxiety better than they expect. Tolerance of anxiety and the frequent concomitant sense of control that comes with knowing one can, in fact, cope while being anxious is a critical outcome of exposure.

Second, your patients need to learn that the feared object (food, their body) is not something that merits their being anxious. As part of this, you want them to learn that the feared outcome (often weight gain) either will not come to pass or is more tolerable (and even beneficial) than expected. Note that you cannot promise your ED patients that they will not gain weight. Some patients will gain weight—indeed, some desperately need to do so. Some patients also will gain sufficient weight that they will move from a societally valued low-weight status to a less-desired middle-weight status or even to a stigmatized high-weight status. For these patients, you will need to identify the feared outcome that drives their fear of weight gain, as well as their beliefs about the tolerability of that feared outcome. Remember that weight gain, taken out of context, is something with ambiguous meaning. Weight gain can be good, bad, or neutral in meaning. Your patients (unless they have ARFID) typically will view weight gain as a profoundly awful thing. You need to know the basis for that extremely negative perception so you can structure exposure in a way that facilitates them learning what they need to learn about weight gain and weight gain tolerance.

ADDITIONAL LEARNING DURING EXPOSURE

In addition to the previous learning, you also want your patients to learn via exposure that they can make effective changes in their lives. In short, you want your patients' learned helplessness to reduce, so they attribute improvements to themselves rather than to the clinician or to random circumstances. This too will enhance a sense of perceived control. Therefore, it is particularly helpful if you reinforce your patients for the positive steps that they have taken, so that they feel inclined and able to make bigger changes and take bigger risks. For example, returning to Chloe in the next session:

> **Clinician:** So, how did you get on with the homework of delaying your exercise when you got the urge?

Chloe: It went so much better than I thought it would. I arranged with my friend that we would take the bus together after I ate my breakfast, so I couldn't go for a run. Riding the bus is super sedentary. Then, I didn't take my running clothes to work, so I couldn't go exercising at lunchtime or after work. I just made sure that I was with people or had something else to do that was sedentary. I wrote down what I was scared of and how scared I was. I was really surprised that I could tolerate my anxiety better than I thought, and the anxiety actually just kept going down. Now, exercising after I eat is just a kind of thought that I don't pay much attention to, and I get on with life. Every now and then, I think that I ought to go for a run, but I think that is just because I don't want to get unfit, so I let myself go for a bit of a jog when I have time and it seems like a fun idea.

Clinician: Now, that is really good to hear. I am not that surprised that the anxiety went down so fast, because that is often what happens when you learn you can tolerate anxiety. Anxiety is a bit like a bully—it gets bigger and more blustery when you are afraid of it, and it tends to creep away when you decide you can handle it. I am glad that you stuck with it so you got to learn. What else have you learned?

Chloe: Well, my weight has really stayed about the same. Maybe because I don't burn up the calories and get so hungry that I binge eat.

Clinician: Great! I want to say that I am really impressed that you came up with some great strategies for stopping your safety behavior of running. That one about eating just before getting on the bus with your friend is genius stuff. You cannot run on the bus, so you can learn to tolerate your anxiety of being sedentary after eating. Similarly, not taking your running clothes with you is a great thought. Well done, you. What do you think should come next?

Chloe: Well, it sounds a bit silly, maybe, but this all started because I was worried that I had eaten regular cream cheese instead of low-fat. I think that I would like to try the regular type next, because I really don't like the low-fat stuff. I know how scary that will be, but I think it is a good idea to deal with that as one of my foods to add in.

Clinician: I like your thinking. A good step. Okay, sounds like you have been going over this in your head, so let's hear your plans . . .

You might think that this is all a bit over the top, offering praise for what looks like a relatively small step that most people would do without thinking about it (delaying exercise; planning a change in eating), but remember how anxious Chloe has been. You will want to offer your patients appropriate positive reinforcement to increase their engagement with exposure. Once your patients are engaged, consider spacing out the praise or saving it for extra efforts; this sort of intermittent reinforcement is more likely to give your patients a stronger sense of agency and resilience. Intermittent reinforcement is also likely to result in the new exposure behaviors being sustained after termination, when your direct praise will no longer be possible.

TREATMENT SETTINGS MATTER

Planning for exposure also needs to consider the treatment setting itself. The setting needs to help your patient experience appropriate levels of anxiety, rather than being very calming and unthreatening. That means that the physical environment should not be designed to be too calming, and you should be prepared to encourage your patients to change, rather than making efforts to calm your patients or exclude them from exposure work (e.g., Meyer, Farrell, Kemp, Blakey, & Deacon, 2014).

Setting Up the Environment for Therapy Sessions

An important objective is not to artificially or deliberately reduce the anxiety-inducing potential of the therapy setting. You should be attentive to the potential for the therapy room to raise your patient's anxiety, allowing you to engage your patient in thinking about feared objects and experience anxiety. For example, many clinicians avoid having weighing scales in the room or tuck them away where their patients cannot see them. Similarly, you might deliberately mask weight charts or behavioral records from your patients as you complete them. As previously noted, this is a short-term way of reducing your patients' anxiety, but one that can lead to greater fear and likelihood of avoidance when your patient finally has to engage with the scales, weight chart, etc.

Even the waiting room can be a valuable source of experiences for your patient that you can use to develop into exposure methods. For example:

> **Billy:** I know that this is the first time that I have been here, but I don't think I should be here at all.
> **Clinician:** Why do you say that?
> **Billy:** I just spent 10 minutes in the waiting room, and everyone else out there looks much sicker than I do. Really, I think I am wasting your time, and you should be getting on with seeing the people who really need help.
> **Clinician:** I am going to ask you to hold onto that thought. My guess is that you are feeling scared that I will say, "There is clearly nothing wrong with you, so please go away"?
> **Billy:** Well, a bit worried about that, of course. Like I said, there are all those sick people out there, after all.
> **Clinician:** Well, I could tell you that is not how it is, but I doubt that would make you believe me, so I am going to say that you are going to have to

sit with that anxiety during the session and see what happens to it while we get on with the assessment. Think you can handle that?
Billy: Well, okay, but it is a pretty big fear.
Clinician: Of course it is. I get that. But let's start with a bit of background to how you came to be here today . . .

Of course, at the end of the session, you should check back on Billy's anxiety level. The exposure to that anxiety should mean that Billy has learned that the anxiety was ill-founded and that he has been able to tell you enough about his ED that he is likely to draw the cognitive conclusion that he really does have a problem. You have also demonstrated to Billy that you don't think it is very important to reduce his anxiety and that you are not distressed by him being anxious. In other words, you have just conveyed the message that it is okay to be anxious.

Intensive Care Settings

Many in- and day-patient units handle the feeding of patients in a relatively cautious way, designed to minimize anxiety (see Chapter 18). This management can manifest as everybody eating the same amount of the same foods, food being weighed precisely by the staff, patients being given choices over their food some days in advance, and the environment being relatively unnatural (e.g., the dining area being a rather somber, quiet room). As noted in Chapter 4, there are times when the aim of feeding is simply to get calories and nutrition into your patients so they can live and think—both of which are prerequisites for successful therapy. This feeding may inadvertently serve as exposure for some lucky patients, but for many it will not. Thus, once the basic conditions of life and ability to think have been met, feeding provides abundant opportunities for exposure and associated learning.

Unfortunately, efforts by clinicians to reduce anxiety in the short-term can mean that patients do not learn to eat in other, more naturalistic environments, such as at home, at work, with friends, etc. Therefore, we recommend that patients in more intensive settings should be encouraged to eat in far less predictable, controlled ways, so that anxiety is elevated enough for them to learn across a range of contexts (e.g., instead of planning meals well in advance, decide at the last minute whether to order take-out pizza or go out to a fast-food eatery).

Weighing Patients in the Treatment Setting

Weighing your patients is an important task in addressing their fears about knowing their weight as well as misunderstandings they may have about the relationship between eating habits and weight (Waller & Mountford, 2015). However, implementing this in some settings is difficult. This can include inpatient units where other staff regard weighing the patient as their role and not one that the clinician should be doing (to which a useful answer is "Given how scared the patient is of being weighed, let's all do it, so that she learns as quickly as possible"). The same applies in many outpatient units, where weighing patients is not carried out (e.g., "Their family doctor is supposed to be doing it and would surely let us know if there is any issue") or where blind weighing is practiced as a matter of policy (Forbush, Richardson, & Bohrer, 2015). Either way, your patients are unlikely to learn that their weight is not out of control (i.e., their feared outcome did not happen), so their anxiety is maintained. In all circumstances, you should be weighing your patient openly, first, to overcome their panic about weight gain being out of control and, second, to allow for effective learning about food not being dangerous (Waller & Mountford, 2015; see Chapter 12 for more detail).

Obviously, many ED clinicians dislike such practices because they wish to avoid feeling that they are a "bad" clinician who raises their patient's anxiety in the short term, even though the result is that they reduce the patient's anxiety longer term. Therefore, you should ensure that supervision addresses the need for using exposure appropriately. To address this barrier, we have found it useful to remind our supervisees (as well as ourselves) of other treatment interventions that involve "short-term pain for long-term gain," such as a course of physical therapy.

"MIXING IT UP"

"Mixing it up" is a term that is useful when explaining effective exposure work to patients. It refers to the idea that we should aim for exposure to include some inherent unpredictability and change, so that our patients do not get into a settled, predictable, and calm routine. To mix it up, we change various aspects of exposure (the types of food, emotion, and body-related behavior that we address; the intensity of the anxiety that we produce; the settings where we ask our patients to try out the changes; etc.) in a relatively unpredictable way. The aim is to maximize speed and generalizability of learning, using the inhibitory learning model (see Chapter 3).

If you use exposure therapy in your clinical work, you are probably used to delivering it in the form of hierarchies. When using hierarchies, many clinicians slowly move their patient nearer to the most feared aspect of the object or situation, in linear steps. For example, in a case of ARFID where Tom fears solid food in case he chokes, you might ask him to start with liquidized food, then move toward more solid food slowly until true solid food is reached.

Slow and steady is not only preferred by clinicians, patients may reinforce you for going slow. Consider the case of Marcy, a patient who fears a wide range of foods as well as eating in front of other people.

> **Clinician:** Now, you have already said that the scariest thing you can imagine is being taken to a restaurant that is a surprise and eating a full meal without knowing what is in it, while other people are with you.

Marcy: You are not going to ask me to do that!! Are you?? I'm not ready.
Clinician: No, of course not, You don't need to worry; I wouldn't do that to you. We won't start with anything that hard. What I want to do is map out a lot of steps along the way.
Marcy: Oh good. That is a big relief.
Clinician: So, you have told me that you are okay with drinking diet drinks and eating undressed salads. So now what we are going to need to do is put the salad and diet drinks at the bottom of the "ladder" and the meal out at the top of it and start working out the steps that go from one to the other. So what would be the next thing up—a bit scary, but not terrifying?
Marcy: I suppose I could manage some fruit by itself next—that is sweet, but not too scary. There is no fat. Then maybe some boiled fish, then chicken with no oil. Plain grilled. Those would be small steps up the ladder . . .
Clinician: Great. We want to keep these steps very doable. So each one should just be a little harder than the one before.
Marcy: I feel so much better now that I know you realize how hard this will be for me.

Although this "low and slow" approach is clearly preferable to Marcy (and likely many other patients, all of whom will reinforce you for adopting it), there are a number of disadvantages to this approach, as we touched on in Chapter 3.

- It is an inherently slow process (as you can see by the number of steps that would still be needed to get Marcy from the chicken to the meal out with friends), keeping the patient ill for longer than necessary.
- It is less likely to generalize, meaning that safety learning occurs only for one food (e.g., potato, but not meat).
- The fear is more likely to be reactivated by other experiences.
- Clinicians vary in how large they make the steps, and how well they stick to advancing through them (Farrell, Deacon, Kemp, Dixon, & Sy, 2013).

It is important to note that experienced exposure therapists have long known that one does not need to follow a hierarchy lock step, meaning that the time that many clinicians take to get to maximal exposure is not necessary. Thus, to get the best outcomes for your patients, you should remember that you are not bound to follow hierarchies of small steps. You might still ask Tom (the previously mentioned patient with ARFID) to rate his feared situations around food in the same way as when creating a hierarchy (indeed, you may still find it useful to build the hierarchy so everything is mapped out), but the pattern of exposure is very different. You would ask Tom to identify the maximum point on the hierarchy where he could start the exposure, and then you should aim to maximize anxiety with later steps. So, in week 1 of exposure, you might identify that he could tolerate eating boiled potato, but in week 2 you might move to a more anxiety-inducing foods (e.g., eating beef jerky). Obviously, Tom needs to be willing to engage in each task. This is where the clinical skill of exposure comes in. Your task is to balance pushing Tom to mix things up and experience significant anxiety, while keeping the tasks in the "doable but very anxiety-provoking" range.

HOMEWORK MATTERS: THE LENGTH OF THE SESSION MIGHT NOT

While it is often suggested that therapy sessions based on exposure should last for more than the standard therapeutic hour (e.g., 90 minutes) to achieve within-session habituation, there is little evidence that this is necessary. Some patients need relatively little time to learn what they need to learn from exposure, whereas others need more time. Thus, the length of a given exposure task will vary based on what it is your patient needs to learn. What is also clear is that repeated practice in a range of settings is critical. Therefore, as you will see from the previous discussion, homework tasks are essential to exposure. This fact should be stressed from the beginning of approaches to EDs that incorporate exposure elements (e.g., CBT, FBT,), as it is important that your patients view therapy as being a full-time occupation (168-hour-a-week therapy), rather than something that is done in 50- or 90-minute slots once per week.

For example, toward the end of her course of CBT, Lisa had achieved a normal body mass index and ceased her restriction and bulimic behaviors. However, she still engaged in body avoidance. She dressed in baggy clothes and avoided mirrors and shopping, in case she saw her reflection in a shop window. Her avoidance maintained her negative body image, making her vulnerable to relapse (Keel, Dorer, Franko, Jackson, & Herzog, 2005), so it was important to address this behavior.

In session 1 of body image exposure, Lisa was treated using mirror exposure. This involved exposure to Lisa's body. She stood in front of a full-length mirror for approximately 40 minutes and monitored the levels of anxiety, negative body perception, and self-esteem. At the end of the exposure, she and her clinician discussed what she had learned and her anxiety about taking part in mirror exposure again. It is valuable to make explicit the change in Lisa's fear expectancies between the beginning and the end of the exposure session (e.g., "I expected that I would be so upset looking at my body in the mirror that I would start sobbing uncontrollably and curl up in a fetal position. What I noticed was that although it was upsetting to look at my body and notice its flaws, I didn't lose control like I thought I would."). Lisa was given homework consisting of

- Repeating the exposure daily in front of a mirror at home;
- Going to local clothes shops and trying on clothes in front of the mirrors in the changing rooms;

- When trying on clothes, make them a mix of baggy and fitting clothes, to vary the context and stimuli of the body exposure; and
- Window-shopping, where she could see her own reflection in the shop windows.

In the second session, Lisa was debriefed about the previous week and described finding that the mirror exposure and wearing more fitting clothes got easier as the week progressed. She was then asked to again undertake mirror exposure in the therapy room with her clinician. She reported that her anxiety was a lot lower at the start of this second session, and it fell very quickly. Most notably, after about 15 minutes of describing her body as she observed it, Lisa said spontaneously that this was becoming "boring" and asked if there was something else that she could be doing. This is always a very positive thing to hear—when your patient is bored, she is not anxious.

To summarize, you should not feel that you need particularly long individual treatment sessions—although different patients need different amounts of time to learn what they need to learn. In addition, you must always treat homework as a very important component of exposure. Further, as with Lisa's case, you should aim to make the exposure as intense as your patient can tolerate, and you should push for change to be "mixed up" rather than slow, steady, and predictable.

COLLABORATION IS KEY

While it is likely to be an obvious point, we will conclude this chapter with one final but critical point. Everything that we have suggested here is dependent on planning exposure work *with* your patients (rather than *for* your patients). Your aim is to work with your patients, because exposure and monitoring its effects need to be personalized. To make exposure effective, you need to be open with your patients from the beginning of therapy about the demands of this approach, as detailed in Chapter 7. Some clinicians see such intense change as being a risk to the therapeutic alliance and thus to treatment outcomes. You should remember that early behavioral change (mostly exposure-based) actually predicts a better therapeutic alliance in CBT (Graves et al., 2017). So remember—being open with your patients about what exposure involves is not likely to scare them off. Rather, the simple process of talking about change can be seen as part of the process of exposure. What is likely more of a problem is when we defer talking about anything that might provoke anxiety in our patients (e.g., delaying raising the topic of weighing), followed by raising such matters later on, when our patients are more likely to feel let down by our having initially misled them.

SUMMARY

Your aim should be to change your patient's response to anxiety via exposure therapy, so that key symptoms are reduced because they are no longer needed as safety behaviors. To summarize, when planning exposure therapy with your patient, you should:

- Consider your patients' everyday lives and how anxiety is generating problems in their eating and body image and plan accordingly.
- Aim to teach your patients via exposure activities that their fears are likely unfounded and that they have the ability to endure their distress, even at higher levels (reinforcing the patient's positive changes).
- For fears that do come true (e.g., progressive weight gain in malnourished patients), your patients will need to learn that they are more tolerable than expected.
- Ensure that the treatment setting is diverse and that neither the environment nor your own concerns limit the diversity of change that will be needed to maximize learning.
- Make the mixture of settings, tasks, intensity, etc. relatively unpredictable ("mixing it up").
- Use homework as a very active part of therapy, stressing the patient's need to undertake exposure in different ways, in different settings.

9

Embarking on Exposure

Important Considerations

When you embark on exposure with your patients, you will need to make a number of decisions. Specifically,

- Will you create a hierarchy of feared stimuli or eschew hierarchies altogether?
- If you decide to organize feared stimuli via the hierarchy method, will you create one hierarchy or several to address different classes of feared situations?
- Regardless of how you organize information about feared situations, how fast will you move through situations, and where will you start?
- What information will you track during exposure to assess whether or not it is working?
- How will you review this information with your patient?
- What will you do if you encounter obstacles?
  - For example, how will you titrate anxiety if the feared situation produces so much anxiety that your patient simply refuses to engage with exposure? Will you strategically use distraction or safety behaviors? Or will you simply switch to an easier situation? Or will you find another way to lessen the intensity of the anxiety (e.g., using a lower calorie version of the same food)?
- How will you teach your patient that exposure is best viewed as a permanent lifestyle strategy for managing anxiety?

You also need to consider how your use of exposure will interact with other strategies included in evidence-based treatments for EDs. For instance, CBT for EDs historically has included the use of delay and alternative strategies to assist patients in resisting the urge to eat or binge eat outside of planned meals and snacks (Fairburn, 2008; Fairburn, Marcus, & Wilson, 1993). Delaying involves "urge surfing" or riding out the urge to binge eat (or vomit, exercise, etc.). Patients using this strategy focus on the urge by observing it instead of trying to make it go away. As a result, they learn that such urges are temporary phenomena that will dissipate in time if they just wait and resist the urge to succumb. The alternative strategy involves engaging in activities that are largely incompatible with eating, vomiting, etc. Taking a bath or shower, talking to a friend, going for a walk (particularly with someone else), or giving oneself a manicure are just a few examples of alternative activities that make it difficult if not impossible to give in to the urge to eat and/or engage in compensatory behaviors. CBT also includes the use of stimulus control strategies to help modulate eating (e.g., getting rid of plates and cutlery when finished eating; limiting binge foods in the home; setting the table formally whenever planning to eat; Fairburn, 2008; Fairburn et al., 1993). While these strategies can be very helpful in changing behavior, in some cases, they may also come to function as safety behaviors or patterns of avoidance and distraction that can interfere with exposure.

The aim of this chapter is to help you think through all of the previously discussed questions and issues. Note that we are not suggesting that you fully abandon the use of the "tried and trusted" strategies from evidence-based treatments. Rather, we suggest that you thoughtfully consider how these and other strategies might help or hinder exposure, so you can make informed decisions collaboratively with your patients. It is important to acknowledge that there are limited empirical data that directly address the many questions raised in the previous (and subsequent) discussion on the treatment of EDs. To the degree possible, we address this lack of data by revisiting the theoretical underpinnings of exposure therapy as well as turning to the existing literature on anxiety disorders. In some cases, we will simply raise questions and consider pros and cons of different clinical choices.

FORCED CONTACT VERSUS EXPOSURE: WHAT IS REALLY HAPPENING?

An important first consideration, which has been briefly raised in earlier chapters, is to correctly determine whether you are or are not actually engaging in exposure therapy. As noted in Chapter 3, there are several types of learning that optimally take place during exposure. More specifically, your patient should optimally learn safety, so that this new learning can compete with fear learning in the future. In addition, your patient needs to learn that she can tolerate fear and other distressing emotions to a greater degree than expected. If exposure is not set up correctly, then this corrective learning will not take place and exposure will likely not work. This is one reason why situations that look like exposure on the surface often fail to teach patients what they need to learn. Many people with anxiety and eating disorders are forcibly exposed to fear producing situations (e.g., via coercion, necessity, inability to escape) to get on with their daily lives. For instance, Dave had panic disorder and was terrified of driving over bridges. However, he was even more terrified of losing his job and ending up homeless. So he drove over a long bridge twice a day, every day to and from work, using safety behaviors and distraction to reduce his anxiety and get through the experience. Although Dave

Embarking on Exposure

was "exposed" to bridges daily, this was not exposure therapy. So remember: **exposure therapy is voluntary and requires the patient to choose to fully experience their anxiety (as well as other potentially distressing emotions) while volitionally foregoing use of safety behaviors and avoidance techniques**.

For an ED example, Astrid was readmitted to a residential treatment center after she failed to maintain weight gained during a previous admission. She reported that although she gained weight during her previous admission, she only ate because she was forced to eat and had no choice. She noted that she played "mental games" to get through her meals and never ate one more bite of food than she was required to eat. Astrid also engaged in covert physical activity whenever she was not being directly observed (shaking her legs, tensing her muscles), and she was convinced that the only reason she did not gain a truly terrifying amount of weight was her continued use of these strategies throughout treatment.

> **Astrid:** Eating makes me so anxious—even after all my treatment. But I had no choice but to eat when I was here before. I hate this place and just wanted to get out—and I definitely didn't want an NG [nasogastric] tube—so I had to eat and just get through it.
>
> **Clinician:** So how did you get through the meals last time?
>
> **Astrid:** I have this place in my head I can go when I don't want to do something. Almost nobody can tell when I do it. I can even have a conversation with my mother when I am there. I got really good at going to my special place in my head while eating last time. Sometimes, though, I can't get there. I don't know why. When that happened, then I just told myself to just get through the meal. Sometimes, I would eat—but chew as little as possible. That way I didn't have to taste the food so much. Swallow it as whole as possible, like a big giant pill. They say food is medicine. Anyway, if you chew less, then some things don't get digested. It sounds gross, but you can see when it comes out and you know you avoided the calories.
>
> **Clinician:** Did you do anything else to get through meals?
>
> **Astrid:** Yeah. There was this one young nurse who sat with us during meals—I think her name was Sandra. If I could get to her table, I could distract myself with the stories she told during meals. You could see that she really hated how bad we felt while eating so she tried to distract us. I would tell myself, "Just listen to Sandra. Don't think about the calories or weight you are going to gain. Just listen to Sandra and remember you can lose it again when you get out." I also burned as many calories as I could even though I wasn't allowed to do real exercise. There are ways around that though . . .

Astrid clearly states that she was not voluntarily engaged in exposure. She utilized both safety behaviors and distraction to tolerate being forced to eat. In this scenario, Astrid is unlikely to learn what she needs to learn to become more comfortable with eating. Many people in the ED field would describe Astrid's experience eating meals during her previous admission as exposure, and they would describe Sandra's job as using exposure. But such eating is better conceptualized as being parallel to Dave's contact with bridges. In both cases, there was forced contact with feared situations, but the necessary features of successful exposure were absent and not a priority. Instead, for Dave, the priority was to simply get through the bridge experience to get to work so he could keep his job. In the case of Astrid, the clinical team's first priority was keeping her alive, but her own first priority was to get out of the unit again. No one's first priority was for Astrid to learn safety and anxiety tolerance.

Even when a patient is barred from using avoidance or safety behaviors, you should be cautious about whether forced contact with exposure stimuli will create an optimal learning experience. A wealth of social psychology literature has demonstrated that when individuals are forced to modify their behavior, they do not experience the subsequent alterations in their beliefs that would otherwise be expected if the behavior change was entirely volitional (e.g., Festinger & Carlsmith, 1959). This is especially pertinent in more intensive care settings, where various program rules often prevent patients from engaging in safety behaviors. To illustrate, it is common in these settings to not allow patients to access a bathroom after eating, to not provide napkins or other things at meals that could be used to hide or manipulate food, and to closely monitor patients to discourage covert exercising behaviors. Although these measures may appear to accomplish "response prevention," they are unlikely to facilitate robust learning. Simply put, your patients must be the agent of their own behavior change to optimize learning from exposure.

It is important to realize that in many ED cases, particularly those with very low weight, patients will have to be forced to eat so they can get adequate nutrition to facilitate both survival and the normalization of cognitive functioning needed for psychotherapy. However, this should not be conceptualized as exposure therapy. Once a patient is out of acute danger, exposure should be introduced (along with a clear rationale as discussed in Chapter 7) so that forced eating becomes "converted" to food exposure. The former is aimed at patient survival, whereas the latter is aimed at patient learning.

This is consistent with treatment for anxiety disorders. Dave's clinician explained the rationale for exposure to Dave. Ultimately, they set up bridge exposure assignments that were deliberately designed to teach Dave both safety learning and fear tolerance. These assignments differed markedly from his daily bridge driving. Then, once Dave had begun to learn fear tolerance and safety learning while driving over the bridge, he and his clinician removed his safety behaviors when driving to work, and Dave agreed to "embrace" his anxiety. In doing so, they converted daily bridge driving to exposure. Similarly, once Astrid was medically safer, she needed start engaging in her eating as exposure therapy. We provide descriptions of specific types of ED exposure in subsequent chapters.

We would be remiss if we did not note that patients can, at times, learn safety even when exposure takes place in less than optimal ways. Examples of this from your patients' lives can be used as powerful examples, supporting the argument for exposure. However, you cannot count on safety and fear tolerance learning spontaneously occurring when contact with feared situations is forced. As such, it is important to distinguish between exposure therapy and forced contact. You may find it helpful to explicitly distinguish these for your patients and their loved ones—otherwise they may think that exposure therapy failed, when, in fact, it was never implemented.

EXPOSURE IN THE CONTEXT OF OTHER THERAPY STRATEGIES

Just as you need to consider the difference between exposure therapy and forced contact, you also need to consider the relationship between exposure and other therapeutic strategies that are components of existing evidence-based treatments for EDs. For instance, and as previously noted, CBT for EDs utilizes a variety of behavioral nonexposure techniques that are used to help ED patients engage in the regular eating that is a foundation of treatment. More specifically, to establish regular eating, patients are taught to formalize their eating (e.g., only eating sitting down in set place when at home), to not combine eating with other activities, to always know in advance what will be eaten for each meal and snack, and to use delays and alternatives to resist eating between planned meals and snacks (Fairburn, 2008). Patients who struggle with feelings of fullness, in early stages of treatment, may be encouraged to wear loose clothing so they cannot scrutinize a "sticking out" stomach or to avoid a sense of their clothing feeling abnormally tight. All of these strategies make sense in the immediate context of helping patients derail chaotic and/or very restrictive eating at the start of treatment.

At the same time, these strategies also may serve as avoidance or safety behaviors and may derail the type of safety learning that you are trying to help your patient experience via exposure. Thus, you cannot assume that regular meals serve as "exposure" when such strategies are being implemented. This does not mean you should abandon the use of these strategies. They may be key, particularly early in treatment, in stabilizing eating, which can provide critical nutrition necessary for improved cognitive, emotional, and physical functioning. Rather, you need to carefully consider the stage of treatment and what you are trying to accomplish. If your goal is, first and foremost, stabilizing eating, then use such strategies when necessary. If your goal is to teach safety learning and anxiety and distress tolerance, then consider ways to eliminate their use, while structuring the nature of the exposure so as to be successful. Naira's treatment illustrates this shift from stabilizing eating to undertaking exposure therapy:

> Naira met criteria for BN. Outside episodes of binge eating, Naira ate only carrots, undressed lettuce leaves, and turkey breast meat. She typically compensated for her binge eating by both vomiting and exercising excessively. At the start of treatment, Naira's clinician pushed her to begin eating three meals and two snacks per day. Initially, this triggered "I've blown my diet, and I am going to get fat" thoughts, and Naira had strong urges to just give up and binge eat. She successfully used alternative strategies and careful meal planning to resist urges to binge eat. She also made sure to always wear very loose clothing so she did not feel any pressure on her abdomen.
>
> After regular eating became more routine for Naira, she and her clinician designed a series of exposure assignments during which Naira was encouraged to experience her anxiety about eating a full meal. For instance, Naira identified her fear expectancy ("I won't be able to tolerate feeling full after eating lunch if I can't distract"), ate her standard lunch, and then attended to her anxiety while sitting in her bedroom. During the planning with her clinician, Naira reported feeling more confident that she could successfully resist the urge to binge eat if she attended to her anxiety in her bedroom as compared to the TV room (which was adjacent to the kitchen) or her kitchen. After several successful exposure trials in her bedroom, Naira moved to the TV room and, ultimately, the kitchen. She and her clinician then added wearing tighter clothing while eating lunch, and Naira recompleted the exposure in each room of her house. Subsequently, she did this while eating out with friends.

TO HIERARCHY OR NOT: THIS IS NOW A QUESTION

For many years, use of fear hierarchies was part and parcel of conducting formal exposure therapy. However, as discussed in earlier chapters, Craske et al.'s (2008, 2014) inhibitory learning model has raised questions about the necessity of using fear hierarchies. More specifically, this model makes a strong case for mixing exposure tasks up and making exposure less predictable. One easy way to do this is to abandon the typical "slow and steady" approach of following the hierarchy systematically and, instead, to introduce exposure tasks in a more random fashion.

Yet there are still good reasons to use or at least build a hierarchy. As noted in several comprehensive reviews (Jacoby & Abramowitz, 2016; Weisman & Rodebaugh, 2018), empirical support for the clinical utility of the inhibitory learning model is still in its infancy. To a large degree, the inhibitory learning model is derived from animal research and other bodies of research investigating learning. Head-to-head comparisons of the clinical application of the inhibitory learning model versus the habituation approach are very limited. To our knowledge, the only comparison of these approaches within an ED paradigm suggested that exposure guided by inhibitory learning principles did not outperform "traditional" exposure aimed at habituation of distress over the course of two sessions (Schyns, van den Akker, Roefs, Hilberath, & Jansen, 2018).

Therefore, hierarchies might still have a place, even if they are not as central as is commonly assumed.

Hierarchies also can be very useful in mapping out the array of feared stimuli and situations that you will encourage your patient to confront. Using a hierarchy to organize a patient's fears does not, a priori, mean that you and your patient have to proceed slowly through the hierarchy in lock-step fashion. Indeed, if you use a hierarchy, we recommend (as noted in Chapter 7):

(a) starting as high up the hierarchy as your patient can tolerate, and
(b) moving through exposure tasks in the hierarchy as swiftly as possible, while increasingly varying the exposure stimuli presented at each fear level.

It is also important to remember that use of hierarchies and the inhibitory learning approach to exposure are not mutually exclusive. For instance, the inhibitory learning model proposes that deepened safety learning can be achieved by combining stimuli and situations for which patients have already completed successful exposure. Nothing in the creation of a hierarchy prevents you and your patients from combining stimuli. Indeed, experienced exposure clinicians have long done this in many cases both with anxiety and ED patients. Shasandra's case illustrates this approach:

> Shasandra's hierarchy of feared eating situations included a wide range of foods and situations, including drinking sweetened iced tea with her best friend, eating two slices of cheese pizza, and eating with a much slimmer friend. Shasandra successfully completed exposure to eating pizza, a highly feared food, in her clinician's office. She also successfully used exposure to learn that she could drink sweetened iced tea with her best friend and resist the urge to exercise afterward. Shasandra's best friend knew about her ED. Together, they decided that Shasandra should try eating pizza and drinking iced tea together at a restaurant that they used to frequent before Shasandra developed her ED. After completing this successfully several times, Shasandra's clinician encouraged them to invite the slimmer friend as well.

Further, although the habituation model did commonly lead to clinicians and patients proceeding up the hierarchy based on the degree to which situations were feared, you can easily jump around in the hierarchy to make exposure less predictable, as per the inhibitory learning model. Moreover, if you want your patient to better tolerate unpredictability, just get him to agree that you can choose the stimuli for in-session exposure and surprise him.

In summary, you have a choice. You can use a hierarchy or not use a hierarchy. If you do use a hierarchy, there are many ways to use it in a way that are consistent with the inhibitory learning approach.

Creating a Hierarchy

Hierarchies are actually quite easy to create. You simply anchor stimuli on both ends of the hierarchy and then fill in the middle steps to create a map that allows you to understand the degree to which your patient fears different situations. Jeremy's case is a classic example:

> **Clinician:** We have discussed your fear of a whole range of foods and eating experiences. So what we are going to do now is put together something called a "hierarchy"—a series of feared events, starting with the least scary and slowly working up to the most scary. Now, you have already said that the scariest thing you can imagine is eating a full serving of cake at that restaurant that specializes in dessert, while your friends share a piece or don't eat dessert at all. On a scale of zero to 100, how much anxiety do you think you would feel doing this? Zero is no anxiety, and 100 is the most intense anxiety you can imagine.
> **Jeremy:** One hundred. I can feel myself shaking just thinking about it. All the calories and what my friends would think of me. They never knew me when I was fat.
> **Clinician:** On the other hand, you have told us that you are okay with drinking black coffee and eating undressed salads or steamed vegetables. Zero to 100—how much anxiety?
> **Jeremy:** Coffee would be zero. The others would be like a 10.
> **Clinician:** Great. So now, what would be a step that is harder than a 10? If you prefer you can also work down. What would be less anxiety-provoking than 100?
> **Jeremy:** I think eating a full serving of regular food—say, dinner at a restaurant when I don't know what is in it—would be really horrible but not as bad as the cake.
> **Clinician:** So, what would you rate it?
> **Jeremy:** Hmmm . . . let's say 90.

The end product is likely to look like Figure 9.1. As previously noted, remember that there is no need to start at the lowest end of the anxiety scale or to work through every item. We also find that it is helpful to omit any mention of quantities of each foodstuff, to avoid calming Jeremy by offering too much predictability.

Because ED patients fear a wide range of foods and eating experiences, you may find it helpful to also have your patients list out all of their feared foods and then have those added into the hierarchy. Remember that once you get patients eating feared foods, you will need to mix up the context. Many ED patients find that eating with other people makes eating a particular food harder or easier. If context markedly influences the intensity of the anxiety experienced for a particular food, you may find it helpful to create subhierarchies to map out the ways in which different circumstances influence predicted anxiety levels.

Anxiety rating	Food to eat
0	Black coffee
10	Undressed salad
10	Steamed vegetables
15	Fruit
20	Crispbread with low-fat spread
30	Bagel with low-fat cream cheese
40	Full-fat milk
50	Creamed potato
50	Chicken burrito
55	Ice cream
60	Full-fat cheese
75	Chips and dips
80	Chocolate
85	Full serving of cake at a regular restaurant
90	Dinner at a restaurant where contents/calories are not known
100	Full serving of cake at a specialist dessert restaurant

Figure 9.1. Example hierarchy of feared foods.

If you choose to create hierarchies, remember that this should be a relatively quick process. You want to move onto starting exposure as soon as possible. Do not delay the process of actually starting exposure by getting "lost in the weeds" of modifying exposure hierarchies, even if your patient indicates a desire to do so. In our experience, when patients communicate such a desire, they may be attempting to avoid exposure, whether purposefully or inadvertently. Remember that the hierarchy need not be overly precise or consist of many small steps. It simply provides a rough map of feared situations and stimuli. As noted in the next section, if your patient completely balks at a given exposure task, there are several ways to titrate anxiety beyond the use of a hierarchy.

TITRATING ANXIETY

Regardless of whether or not you use hierarchies, it will be important to consider the myriad ways that you can adjust anxiety and other distressing emotions and sensations so as to create exposure assignments that are both challenging and manageable. You want your patient to improve as fast as possible, and that will only happen by encouraging her to face her anxiety. At the same time, exposure should provide the opportunity for safety learning and improved distress tolerance—which means it should cause significant distress, but not so much distress that the patient flees from the experience. Having a good understanding of how to titrate anxiety and other distressing experiences will help you manage this challenging task.

Start With Moderately Challenging Situations

One easy way to titrate anxiety is simply to start by choosing situations that your patient expects will cause a moderate amount of anxiety (say a 50 on a scale of zero to 100). You can then observe to what degree your patient truly found the exposure challenging, based on both self-report and behavioral indicators of distress. If 50 was distressing but clearly quite manageable, simply encourage your patient to begin incorporating all exposure activities listed below 50 into his lifestyle (you may need to help him with some planning for some tasks) and start working on items that were rated as more difficult than 50. In fact, once you identify the level at which you want to start exposure, you can simply assign your patient to eat all the lower-level items on a more regular basis. In the case of Jeremy, he and his clinician decided to start exposure with a chicken burrito. His clinician also asked him to just start incorporating all the foods below a 50 into his diet on a more regular basis. Jeremy was already eating undressed salad, steamed vegetables, and fruit. But he was not regularly eating the other mildly anxiety-provoking foods on the hierarchy. Jeremy reported it took some effort to start eating the other foods but did not find it terribly anxiety-provoking and was successful.

Intensifying Exposure as Needed

You certainly do not need to wait to increase the intensity of exposure if the original task was more manageable for your patient than expected. Skillful exposure clinicians are adept at utilizing subtle strategies during exposure to intensify distress as necessary. While the particular strategy that you use will likely be based on the nature of the exposure task, from a broad perspective, these intensification strategies will involve having your patient interact with her feared stimuli to a greater (and more distressing) extent than the current exposure task is creating. Consider the example of Alexandra, who began an exposure session with her clinician, viewing her body in a mirror while wearing a form-fitting leotard.

> **Alexandra:** I'm really surprised that I'm not as anxious as I thought I'd be. When we were preparing to do this, I doubted whether I could go ahead without crying and shaking. This honestly isn't half as bad as I thought.
> **Clinician:** It's great that your experience has been positive thus far. This happens occasionally where we anticipate something to be more difficult than it really is. How would you rate the intensity of your distress right now?
> **Alexandra:** Only about a 30 or 35. Before we started, I thought this would be a 70!

Clinician: I'm happy that you've had this pleasant surprise. Given what we've discussed previously about the need for exposure to be as challenging as possible to maximize your benefit, I'm wondering if we can put our heads together to figure out how to make this more challenging for you?

Alexandra: Okay. What did you have in mind?

Clinician: Well, I remember that you described one of your safety behaviors when wearing tight-fitting clothing like this was to "suck in" your tummy to try giving off the appearance of it being flat. I can see you're not doing that right now, but I'm wondering if you can try allowing your tummy to "stick out?" Can you try pushing it out?

Alexandra: Sure, I can try if you think it'll help (*pushes out tummy*). Hmm, this does make me more anxious. I really don't like the way it looks when it protrudes so much—like there's a volleyball under this leotard.

Clinician: I appreciate your willingness to try it. How distressing is it now?

Alexandra: Quite a bit more. I'd say 60.

Clinician: Okay. I would certainly understand your preference to continue the exposure at the lower distress level, but I don't think that will benefit you much in the long term. I'm going to encourage you to carry on this exposure while trying to keep your tummy protruding.

Other examples of how to intensify the experience of exposure are going to be case-dependent. For example, a patient with ARFID might be asked to feel the avoided food with their fingers, and to describe the experience in great detail, prior to eating it.

Strategic Use of Avoidance/Distraction and Safety Behaviors

Just as there are circumstances when distress needs to be increased during exposure, there are also circumstances, albeit more infrequent, when distress may need to be temporarily decreased during exposure. This may be needed if your patient *genuinely* appears to be incapable of tolerating the current level of distress. For example, a patient may become so intensely distressed that he immediately gets up and declares an intention to terminate the session (and perhaps therapy altogether). Fortunately, in our experience, these sorts of circumstances are relatively rare. Indeed, we have had patients who were so anxious that they reported their anxiety was at 100 on their first exposure, and they still got through the experience and benefited. On the rare occasions in which patients find exposure intolerable, these tend to occur early in the course of treatment before the patient has developed sufficient confidence that they can endure their elevated distress. Nonetheless, these circumstances do occur occasionally and warrant your consideration of strategic use of safety behaviors or other avoidance/distraction techniques to titrate the anxiety to a lower level. Some authors have posited that using a gradual, "fading" approach to safety behaviors versus encouraging their immediate elimination may make exposure therapy more acceptable to patients without diminishing its effectiveness (Rachman, Radomsky, & Shafran, 2008), although the evidence for this is mixed (Bowie, Jones, & Stobie, 2016).

If you do elect to allow your patient to engage in some safety behaviors during exposure, we suggest proceeding with the following suggestions in mind:

- Encourage your patient to minimize their use of the safety behavior as much as they possibly can during and after exposure. Ideally, your patient will agree to use their safety behaviors with considerably less frequency than is typical for them.
- Be clear with your patient that further exposure will be needed *without* the reliance on safety behaviors or other avoidance/distraction to manage their distress. True safety learning cannot occur in the context of "artificial safety."
- Carefully assess what your patient reports learning from their exposure activities, paying particular attention to how your patient attributes the nonoccurrence of her feared outcomes. Many patients misattribute the nonoccurrence of their feared outcomes to their own safety behaviors (e.g., "I didn't gain a bunch of weight, but I think it's because I chewed the food very slowly").

Special Considerations for Self-Injuring Patients

The previously discussed considerations regarding strategic use of safety behaviors and other avoidance/distraction may be especially important when using exposure therapy with patients who use self-injurious behaviors to regulate their emotional distress. Given that your patient's safety must be of the utmost priority, use of exposure to temporarily induce negative emotions among individuals who respond to negative emotions with self-injury must be handled with some caution. As a general rule of thumb, it is important to be closely in tune with how your self-injuring patient is responding to the distress that is evoked by exposure. Open, direct dialogue about the propensity or actual occurrence of self-injurious behavior is critical. You should also consider whether any propensity toward self-harm is actually worsened by the exposure work, or whether the level simply remains as it was before the exposure is used. To the degree exposure helps patients feel more in control and teaches distress tolerance, it can also lead to improvements in desire to self-injure.

For patients who do demonstrate difficulty with refraining from self-injury in the context of exposure activities, depending on the nature of the self-injury, you may consider utilizing the previously described de-intensifying strategies (as well as choosing to start at a lower place in the hierarchy) as a means to build confidence and mastery that the distress can be endured without any self-injury. You may also find it helpful to develop a clear plan for what your patients will do after the exposure is finished. This plan can reduce the chance of needing to decide what to do when in a heightened state of arousal. Finally, in the event that your patient is engaging in self-injury to either an unacceptably high consistency or degree of risk, you may consider postponing exposure work until your patient can develop the improved emotion regulation skills necessary to proceed with exposure. This general strategy has been utilized to good effect in other similar clinical populations, such as individuals with comorbid borderline personality disorder and PTSD (e.g., Harned, Korslund, Foa, & Linehan, 2012).

EXPOSURE AS A LIFESTYLE

Our last section of this chapter may be the most important. When embarking on exposure therapy, you can increase the likelihood of a successful outcome for your patient if you take time to explain the benefits of conducting "lifestyle exposure," in addition to the systematic exposure activities that typically occur either within therapy sessions or between therapy sessions as planned homework. Put simply, exposure will be more effective the more that your patient adopts it as a new mindset when faced with anxiety-evoking scenarios. Although the planned exposure activities that occur within and between therapy sessions are undoubtedly beneficial, your patients will benefit substantially further from "wearing their exposure hat" at every opportunity that presents. In other words, you should encourage your patients to view the "silver lining" in their unplanned anxieties that arise throughout the week as rich opportunities to experience further safety learning. Consider the following dialogue between James and his clinician.

> **Clinician:** Okay, James, I think we have a good plan for your exposure homework during the week ahead. Let's move to discussing a related topic—something we refer to as "lifestyle exposure."
> **James:** What is that? It sounds a little weird.
> **Clinician:** Lifestyle exposure refers to the idea that, in addition to all of the planned exposures we'll do together in our sessions and you'll do for homework during the week, you will get further benefit from using unplanned stressors that occur during the week as opportunities for exposure. This means that you will get past your problem faster if you go out each day looking for opportunities to make yourself anxious and face your fears. These opportunities can and should go beyond the exposure homework we've planned. What are your thoughts as you're hearing me describe this?
> **James:** Um, I think I understand. Basically, I've got to say, "Come on anxiety, give me your best shot," and try to find ways to challenge myself.
> **Clinician:** Exactly. You've got it. So, do you have any ideas for how you can accomplish this?

James: Well, we already planned for me to eat a lot of foods this week that I'm worried about choking on. Scrambled eggs, tuna salad, and pasta are all foods I'm going to try. One idea I have is looking for ways I can make myself more anxious when trying these foods. For example, if the break room at my work gets too crowded, I usually stop eating and leave because having more people there makes me more worried I'll choke. So I could try to eat at times when there are more people in the break room and maybe even sit at a table with some coworkers. They won't be expecting that from me!

Clinician: Excellent idea. Adopting this mindset where you are looking for ways to further face your fears and choosing to be anxious will help you get the most out of treatment.

James' clinician helped him begin to consider ways that he could be opportunistic and capitalize on typical stressors as a means of increasing his overall "dosage" of safety learning. Helping James begin to think in this way may stimulate further recognition of opportunities for lifestyle exposure. For example, James may recognize that his slow eating pace and excessive chewing are safety behaviors aimed at minimizing the likelihood of choking and decide to push himself to eat at a faster pace with less chewing before swallowing. The more that James intertwines exposure principles into his lifestyle, the more variation there will be in his safety learning, thereby increasing the accessibility of this learning in future instances when he confronts his fears. The moral of the story here is that you should make every effort to encourage your patients to take exposure work beyond planned assignments and into a new way of going about responding to fear in their day-to-day living.

SUMMARY

The aim of this chapter was to help you think through some of the nuts and bolts of doing exposure. As an exposure clinician, you have many choices to make throughout the therapy process. Hopefully, you now have a good roadmap for navigating the big picture decisions and can apply that to the many different types of exposure we will discuss in Part 3 of this book.

Summary points—Part 2: Preparing for Implementation of Exposure Therapy

- Begin with a functional assessment of your patient's fears and behaviors, so that you can understand their avoidant and safety behaviors and plan their exposure therapy to address those individual functions.
- Such a functional analysis should include the role of family and others in responding to and accommodating the avoidant and safety behaviors.
- You should explain exposure therapy to your patient but also allow that you might have to explain it again as you change therapy targets.
- Plan exposure collaboratively with the patient and make it fit their wider life.
- To enhance learning, "mix it up," ensuring that you combine contexts and approaches and ensure that there is unpredictability in exposure activities.
- Be prepared for the practicalities of exposure work, so that you are ready when you start implementing it as you move into the next part of the book.

PART 3

Applying Exposure to Different Eating Disorder Problem Areas

In this section of the book, you will learn how to use exposure therapy to address specific aspects of eating disorders (EDs) for which anxiety commonly plays a key maintaining role. In each case, it will be clear that these aspects of EDs are relatively transdiagnostic features and symptoms. As such, you will see that exposure can be applied across a wide range of ED diagnoses and to patients of all ages. We also outline steps in troubleshooting that you will need to address roadblocks that result from the patient's pathology, the situation, or your own concerns.

10

Exposure to Food and Eating

Alongside body image disturbance (see Chapter 13), anxiety over food and eating is a core defining characteristic of (EDs) such as AN and BN among adults and adolescents and is central to many cases of ARFID. Food- and eating-related anxiety often stems from fear of uncontrollable weight gain (Waller & Mountford, 2015) or loss of control over eating (e.g., binge eating). However, in some cases (particularly ARFID), the emotional reaction is about other issues (e.g., disgust or fear of choking).

These fears are going to be at the heart of your work with ED patients, regardless of your profession. We all should be discussing food with our patients. Thus, whether you are a dietitian (see the following example), nurse, therapist, or physician, you will need to work with your patients to change their eating patterns. Moreover, you will need to help your patients make this work in a wide variety of settings and contexts.

We recognize that professions and professionals vary in their focus when it comes to food and eating and have different levels of knowledge about food and nutrition (e.g., Cordery & Waller, 2006). For example, if you are a dietitian, you might be trying to get your patient to eat a more balanced diet, whereas if you are a physician, you might be mostly interested in persuading them to eat more carbohydrates to enhance their serotonin levels. A nurse, in contrast, might want to get his patient to socialize over meals with other patients, and a therapist might want to stabilize her patient's eating to get them ready to move onto behavioral experiments. Each of these goals is valid and potentially useful, but in each case the clinician is going to have to start the process with overcoming the patient's anxiety about introducing a new food or about starting to eat differently. That means that, regardless of the profession to which you belong, you often will need to use exposure as Step 1.

Food and eating exposure will be structured and paced differently based on the nature of the ED, as well as your patient's specific learning history (both prior to and following the development of the eating problem). The overarching goal is to create a scenario in which your patient can learn what she needs to learn with respect to eating, food, and feared outcomes. It is important to remember that you need to ferret out why your patient fears something to structure exposure properly. For instance, one patient might fear pizza because she thinks it will trigger a binge, another patient might fear pizza because she is concerned it will lead to weight gain, a third patient might fear pizza because he is worried he will choke on it, and yet another patient may fear the pizza because the pizza is made with artificial ingredients and is therefore not "clean and healthy." If you were to set up exposure assignments for each of these four patients, exposure would look different. Indeed, for some of these patient examples, you might not even start exposure using pizza because another food would work better.

In the following discussion, we provide three specific examples of food exposure. These examples include fear of specific "binge foods," fear of food causing uncontrollable weight gain, and fear of the process of eating. In each case, we use the principles outlined in previous chapters to engage patients in changing their avoidance of the feared object.

FEAR OF "BINGE FOODS"

> Jenny is a 35-year-old woman with a long-standing history of BN. She has a strong fear of specific foods, which she calls "binge foods," because she is used to bingeing immediately after eating them. She avoids them for as long as she can, but the lack of carbohydrates in the rest of her diet makes it more likely that she will binge on those foods, reinforcing the idea of a "binge food."

In the following dialogue, Jenny's clinician, who is a dietitian, introduces Jenny to the idea of food exposure. During this process she also makes sure to identify Jenny's feared outcomes.

Clinician: Looking at your diary, what is clear is that you are eating almost no carbohydrates as part of your normal eating pattern. Then you binge on cookies, chocolate, and candy in the evening.

Jenny: Yes, so you see why I call them "binge foods"—they make me binge whenever I eat them.

Clinician: Well, if we look at your eating pattern, there is another interpretation—that you binge on those high-carbohydrate foods because you have starved yourself of carbs all day, and your body is craving them. So if you were to start the day with some carbohydrate—say, a bagel—then that might mean that your needs were lower later in the day and you would be able to resist the urge to binge.

Jenny: But something like a bagel at breakfast? I would be too scared that I would binge immediately and then binge lots more in the day.

Clinician: So your fear is that you would not be able to keep from bingeing after you ate a bagel, right?

Jenny: Exactly. And I worry that I'll just carry on bingeing.

Clinician: Well, it is certainly possible that you would get into a cycle of binges if you let yourself binge straight away. But what happens when you perpetually avoid carbs?

Jenny: I wind up bingeing on them anyway.

Clinician: So to avoid your fear of binge eating uncontrollably, which you think will be triggered by carbs, you avoid carbs. This reduces your anxiety, but it also makes you crave carbs. And when you finally give in, you binge.

Jenny: So how do I ever get past this? Sounds impossible.

Clinician: I think that the best way of finding out would be to try it and see. If you can eat the bagel and learn that you actually can tolerate your anxiety about the possibility of bingeing, you might learn that you are tougher than you think. In other words, I think we need to do that "exposure" thing that we were talking about.

Jenny: A whole bagel, though?

Clinician: Well, you could build up very slowly—eat a tiny bit of a bagel on Day 1, then a slightly bigger bit on Day 2, and so on. How long do you think that would take?

Jenny: A really long time.

Clinician: So let's figure out an amount that seems doable but still raises your anxiety quite a bit about the possibility of bingeing. We want you to really learn something here. I should note that you could do all that in one step, so that you can learn more quickly that other foods are not "binge foods" either. It depends how long you want this to take.

Jenny: So could I try one bagel on one day, see if I can cope with that, and then decide from there?

Clinician: Definitely, though if you are going to do that. I would make it tomorrow, because if it works, then you can try it a few more times in the week—every day would be good. Also, the longer you put this off, the more your anticipatory anxiety will grow, and that will make it harder to do.

Jenny: I could see that.

Clinician: And later, as you gain more practice with this, you can also learn to eat that way in different places, different types of bagel, and so on. But let's nail down what this exposure will look like tomorrow.

Jenny: Okay.

Clinician: So just to make sure we are on the same page. Exactly what do you fear will happen if you eat the bagel? We could call this your fear prediction.

Jenny: I fear I will lose control and binge after eating the bagel and will just binge all day long.

Clinician: So you fear you won't be able to keep from binge eating, which you predict will come with eating a bagel?

Jenny: Yes.

Clinician: Do you think the urge to binge will fade over time? Or will it just go on and on?

Jenny: That is also what I fear. I fear the urge will just be there and get bigger and bigger and bigger, and I will eventually give in.

In Jenny's case, you will notice that the object of fear is the food and its potential to trigger uncontrollable binges, rather than the eating process itself. This is a classic pattern where you can use exposure. In the previous example, Jenny's dietitian makes sure that Jenny's fear predictions are fully articulated. By doing this, the dietitian increases the probability that Jenny will experience a violation of her expectancy (i.e., her expectation that she will binge) because she is attending to it. In the following dialogue, the dietitian helps Jenny figure out how to structure the actual exposure. The aim is to make sure that Jenny will experience quite significant (but manageable) anxiety, attend to her expectancy (i.e., fear prediction that she will binge), and discover that her expectancy does not come to pass or is not as bad as predicted. In Jenny's case, optimally she will not binge. So the dietitian looks to create a situation that both triggers anxiety *and* facilitates Jenny's attempts to resist binge eating. You can think of this as creating steps on a hierarchy, although Jenny's dietitian does not formally do this.

Clinician: Do you fear you won't be able to keep yourself from bingeing even if we make it a bit harder to binge?

Jenny: What do you mean?

Clinician: Well, I imagine that some situations will make it harder to resist binge eating and some easier. For example, you typically binge in the kitchen. What if you went to a bagel shop, ordered one bagel, and then ate it outside in the park? Does that still seem difficult? How would that compare to trying to eat a bagel in your kitchen surrounded by cookies and chocolate?

Jenny: Those are very different. I really, really, really think I would binge in my kitchen surrounded by cookies and chocolates. But a bagel from the shop in a park? That seems less scary but still scary. I mean I still fear that eating the bagel could trigger a binge because *I could* go back into the shop and buy a bunch of bagels if I gave in. But that would require buying the bagels while a lot of people looked at me, wondering why one person needed so many bagels. So while I am very anxious about eating a bagel tomorrow morning, even in the park, because I am scared I will binge and lose control, it does seem more manageable than trying to do this in my kitchen with lots of sweets around.

Dietitian: Okay, so let's nail down exactly what you are going to do tomorrow.

Jenny: I am going to go to the bagel shop tomorrow morning and buy a bagel for my breakfast. I am going to eat it in the park.

Dietitian: Great. What time do you plan to do this?

Jenny: Hmmm. . . . Let's say 7 AM because I need to be at work at 8:30. And I think I need some time between when I eat the bagel and when I have to work with people if you want me to focus on my anxiety.

Dietitian: Excellent. Are you going to bring your work stuff with you, or will you need to go home again?

Jenny: I can bring my work stuff with me and go straight to work.

Dietitian: Perfect. Now when you eat the bagel and after you eat the bagel, I want you to really allow yourself to experience your anxiety about the possibility of binge eating.

Jenny: Should I read a magazine or do my nails to stop myself thinking about bingeing?

Dietitian: We can think of those as sort of safety behaviors that you use in really tricky situations where the primary goal is simply to not binge. However, here, when we are doing exposure, the aim is somewhat different. You want to experience your anxiety so you can learn that you can tolerate it. You also want to really test out your fear prediction that you can't eat any carbs without binge eating. So let's not use those safety behaviors.

As discussed in Chapter 9, you need to distinguish between doing exposure, which is designed to facilitate inhibitory learning, and helping your patients do things that need to happen in their daily lives even if they do not learn anything about their harm expectancies from the experience. For instance, Jenny's dietitian had taught her to use the related strategies of delaying a binge and doing something pleasurable instead of bingeing to help Jenny reduce her binge eating in everyday life. It is possible that simply by delaying a binge, Jenny *might* learn something about her harm expectancy that could inhibit her fear in the future. In other words, this could serve as inadvertent exposure. But it is just as possible that she might simply learn a safety behavior that helps her decrease bingeing without learning she can tolerate anxiety. The exposure task, in contrast, is explicitly set up in a way to maximize inhibitory learning.

As raised previously, you also need to encourage your patients to maximize the speed and diversity of change. So, you will want to try to avoid very slow graded exposure, with its slow progression through hierarchies ("a bit more bagel"), unless it is the only way possible. However, as previously demonstrated, you will still want to titrate the exposure to create anxiety that is manageable so that your patient can learn what she needs to learn. Over time, Jenny progressed to eating a wide variety of bagels, with and without cream cheese or butter, in a wide variety of settings—including her kitchen. She also ate by herself and with other people so as to further vary context and layer different fear-provoking situations (Jenny also feared other people seeing her eat anything but salad).

FEAR OF UNCONTROLLABLE WEIGHT GAIN

The other most commonly feared consequence of food is that it will result in massively disproportionate, uncontrollable weight gain. You will be used to patients who believe strongly that eating even a single bite of "forbidden" or "feared" food will result in their weight going up and continuing to do so. The fact that this is "magical thinking" does not stop it from being a very powerful maintaining factor in EDs.

> Sally's ED started when she was 15 after she decided she needed to be very slim to be a better diver. Sally described herself at 15 as "too curvy, almost a little chubby; I still had baby fat combined with big boobs." Since then she has alternated between periods of intense dietary restriction, which result in weight loss, and periods of intermittent binge eating, which result in weight gain. Sally reports that she hasn't eaten bread in years—even during her periods of binge eating. She states, "If I ate it, I know that my weight would start going up, and that it would keep on going up even if I stopped eating bread straightaway."

Addressing Sally's fear involves two components—getting her to start eating her feared food and then getting her to continue eating it. In each case, you will use exposure to treat her anxiety. This is also an example of how we are more likely to be effective if we consider maintaining factors than if we try to uncover how the fear developed in the first place. Sally is no longer a diver, so focusing on why she started restricting is not helpful. Further, unlike fears relating to a specific experience (see Matthew's case in the following discussion), fear of uncontrollable weight gain can be a multicausal phenomenon in your patient's development (e.g., a number of specific experiences including comments by a diving coach, reading magazines over several years, changes during puberty, teasing by peers, transmission of weight stigma from family members and society at large). This means that when you work with Sally, you should start by focusing on the here-and-now nature of the fear.

You will also need to consider her biological state, specifically as it relates to the appropriateness of her current weight. If she is not underweight, then weight stability is not an important short-term target. However, if she is underweight, then weight gain is an important clinical goal for your exposure work. In this case, let us assume Sally is underweight, and while she is not currently losing weight, she is maintaining an unhealthily low body mass index of 17, which is resulting in both physical sequelae (e.g., loss of menses, decreased bone density) and numerous fights with her partner. In short, Sally's fear of uncontrollable weight gain needs to be addressed in the context of her need for actual weight gain. Therefore, it is the fear of uncontrollability (and the predicted never-ending weight gain) that is the target of the exposure work with her therapist.

Note that Sally does not have a history of ever living in a higher weight body (even though she felt she was slightly "curvy and chubby" at 15). Although you cannot know for sure where her weight will end up once her eating normalizes, it is unlikely she will gain a socially stigmatizing amount of weight—particularly since her binge episodes result in relatively small, transitory amounts of weight gain. However, if Sally was at a quite high weight before the start of her ED and it appeared likely she would end up at a weight that would lead to weight stigma from society (e.g., if her family members' bodies were all higher weights and this appears to be her family's genetic body type), then you would potentially focus on the fear of being able to tolerate the socially stigmatizing higher weight given that it is likely she will gain a significant amount of weight and it may be somewhat "uncontrollable." In Sally's case, however, it appears likely she will simply end up with a socially acceptable body weight based on her own medical history and her description of her family's body type.

One other consideration in conducting exposure to fear of uncontrollable weight gain is the degree to which your patient is in treatment voluntarily. In the following scenario, Sally is in voluntary outpatient treatment, which she initiated on her own, albeit with encouragement from her partner. Sally is ambivalent about treatment and against gaining weight, but she also can choose to engage in exposure if presented with a compelling enough rationale. Moreover, she is in a position to choose to experience her anxiety and stop her safety behaviors. As noted in Chapter 9, extremely low-weight ED patients in inpatient care often have largely ceded (or been forced to cede) control over their care to hospital staff, and treatment may feel (and even be) quite involuntary. Under these conditions, weight gain is likely to be experienced as very uncontrollable, and patients will liberally engage in safety behaviors (including covert ones you cannot see) to tolerate the anxiety associated with mandated eating and weight gain. For these patients, weight gain also may confirm, not violate, harm expectancies (Murray et al., 2016). In cases like these, you will often want to see a certain amount of weight stabilization and normalization of eating (and cognitive function) prior to embarking on exposure; you need your patient to move from less voluntary care to a somewhat more voluntary, active, and collaborative stance. This will better set the stage for successful exposure.

> **Clinician:** So, however your fear about bread developed, it is going to be important to work with that fear as it is now. So let's break it into two parts, rather than thinking about it all as one. First, you are terrified that even small amounts of bread are going to have a big effect on your weight. Is that right?
> **Sally:** Yes, that is why I cannot eat it at all.
> **Clinician:** I may be mistaken here, but it also sounds like you think you cannot tolerate any weight gain.
> **Sally:** Totally. There is no way I will be able to stand being any fatter than I already am right now. Not even a tiny bit. I want to be thinner, not bigger.

Clinician: And then, second, you worry that if you ate bread even once, your weight would keep going up and up and up, and you could never get it to stay stable.

Sally: Well, of course. It's like a slippery slope—once my weight starts going up, I won't ever be able to stop, and I will just end up as a serious fatso.

Clinician: So let's start with that first fear prediction—that eating even a small amount of bread is going to make your weight shoot up and you won't be able to tolerate it. The important bit is not how much weight precisely, but whether your fear comes true. So, it looks like what we will need you to do is to try eating differently for a week or even two and see whether or your fear prediction comes true. Does your weight shoot up massively when you eat any bread, and are you unable to tolerate even a small amount of weight gain? During this time, you will also have the chance to practice tolerating your anxiety.

Sally: What about how much my weight will go up by?

Clinician: The amount is not so important right now—we will come back to that when we talk about something called "behavioral experiments." For now, we just need to see if the bread has a big intolerable effect on your weight and give you a chance to practice tolerating your anxiety about weight gain.

Sally: So, what would that look like? It sounds terrifying . . .

Clinician: We'll start by cutting out your avoidance. To cut out the avoidance, we would need you to take the risk of eating something bread-based—say, a slice of toast at breakfast each day in addition to the egg white omelet you currently eat. Then it would be important not to use any of your safety behaviors, like exercising, so that you can learn something about your fear prediction and learn to better tolerate your anxiety about weight gain. Paradoxically, the better you get at tolerating anxiety, the less it seems to matter.

This test of a small (but not tiny) amount of bread on a daily basis offers a good opportunity to test out Sally's fear prediction. In all likelihood, she will not gain a lot of weight. Indeed, she very well may not gain any, and her harm expectancy will be violated. Sally did eat the bread and found over 2 weeks that she did not gain a meaningful amount of weight. Importantly, because Sally and her therapist had been regularly weighing her (see Chapter 12), Sally had plenty of data that she could use see if her weight actually changed.

However, this will not be enough in Sally's case. While our approach would be sufficient if she did not actually need to gain weight, more is needed to address Sally's fear of the *uncontrollability* of weight gain, given that Sally needs to eat enough to actually gain weight. Further, this next element also may need to be addressed before patients like Sally will even agree to change their eating, because the fear of uncontrollability can stop patients from even trying to change. After all, would you let go of a rope while dangling off a rock face if you had no faith that gravity's effects could be countered another way? Therefore, you may need to plan the exposure with Sally so that it addresses *both* her fear of weight gain *and* her fear of uncontrollability. Let's continue with our scenario.

Sally: But wait a minute. Suppose I did that—what if my weight *did* go up? Once it starts, I won't be able to stop it even if I stop eating bread. I am not going back to being a little on the chubby side! I am much better like this.

Clinician: There are two things there, so let's unpackage that. First, your anxiety is making you think in a very black-and-white way—either your weight stays where you are *or* you will be significantly overweight. I think that it is possible that when you are less anxious you will be more able to see the possibility of something in between—that more flexible thinking is much easier when you are less starved and less anxious.

Sally: Okay, that makes sense, given that educational material that you gave me. But what was the second thing?

Clinician: The second thing is that you are seriously underweight, and your life is suffering as a result—decreasing bone density and loss of your period, angry partner, unable to get pregnant, scared parents, nagging friends. So, if you want your life back, you are going to need to gain *some* weight. The real issue is not "staying where I am is better than being overweight" but "can we get you back to a healthy weight that works for you, without it going on to indefinitely gain weight?"

Sally: Is that even possible? And how do I know that it is going to work for me? I might still overshoot and end up like I used to be . . .

Clinician: Well, let's start where we were—you need to eat more at first to learn that you can tolerate the anxiety associated with eating and possible initial weight gain. Then you would need to eat more than that so that you weight goes up to a more healthy level, but in a controllable way. That way you will be able to see whether your fear prediction about never-ending, uncontrollable weight really comes to pass.

Sally: Okay, I see that, but what if it wasn't controllable and shot up?

Clinician: The next stage might sound a bit odd, but bear with me. Next, you will need to learn to *stop* gaining weight.

Sally: You mean it is two things to learn? How to gain weight and how to stop gaining weight?

Clinician: Exactly. So, what I am going to suggest is that you start for now by eating a bit more bread and not compensating with exercise so you will overcome your avoidance and safety behaviors. Then you will learn that you can tolerate the anxiety, and you can test your fear prediction that even a tiny amount of bread will cause your weight to shoot up. After that, you eat more bread and other things, so that your weight does actually go up a bit. Then cut back on your eating a little, so that your weight stabilizes. Then you go back to eating more to gain weight deliberately for a few weeks, then you stabilize again, and so forth. That way, you are learning that your eating and weight are controllable to some degree and that when you get back to a healthy weight, you already know that you can stop. It will take several weeks, but the benefit about doing necessary weight gain in this "stepped" manner is that you learn that you can tolerate both anxiety and controlled weight gain, regardless of whether you are thinking about gaining weight or about gaining weight uncontrollably.

Our experience of using this approach with underweight patients is that it reduces anxiety at all levels, by making the process of weight gain predictable and controllable enough for them to be willing to engage in exposure (after all, exposure will not work if your patient simply refuses to try it). This is often the case even from the outset, because the plan to "stage" weight gain and weight stability is somewhat reassuring to patients. This graded approach to exposure also is one where you will find that you can change the plan as you proceed. For example, we routinely find that patients describe the process of gain/stabilize to be "boring" after two or three cycles, as they now know that they can stop weight gain now if they want to and believe that they will be able to at a later stage, when they are approaching a healthy, functional weight. When you hear that the overall process of weight gain has become boring to the patient, you should know that you have used exposure effectively, as "boring" and "anxious" are not terribly compatible.

As noted earlier, patients who are extremely malnourished and at extremely low weights will likely need to have some degree of weight stabilization occur before you start exposure. The case of Sally, however, shows how you can use exposure to address fear of weight gain in patients who are low weight but relatively medically stable. Note that if your patient does completely refuse to engage in weight gain exposure, you can experimentally try to reduce that anxiety using imaginal exposure (see Chapter 13 for a brief example of imaginal exposure for body image concerns and Chapter 15 for more in-depth discussion).

FEAR OF EATING

In the previously discussed case examples, the fear focused on the negative effects that the foods themselves would have on the individual. In other cases, it is the actual experience of eating that is more central to the patient's fear. For example, Matthew is a young man with ARFID who is being treated by his family physician.

Exposure to Food and Eating

In his case, the texture of food evokes strong anxiety, making his eating pattern very limited:

> **Matthew:** I just can't eat solid foods. I can feel them as a lump in my throat, and I start to panic that I am going to choke again. Even thinking about this makes me feel like my throat is closing and I might choke.
> **Clinician:** Well, it sounds like your avoidance of eating solid foods never allows you to learn whether or not you'd choke, so you stay worried and it gets worse.
> **Matthew:** I suppose it does get worse—I used to eat some things that were a bit solid, like very well-boiled potatoes. I never choked on them—they were very soft—but I started to worry that I might, so I cut them out too...
> **Clinician:** So you avoid ever getting anxious by cutting out more and more foods?
> **Matthew:** Yes. It just felt safer that way. And now people are noticing, so I am avoiding them in case they try to push me to eat scary things.
> **Clinician:** That is usually the pattern once you start avoiding. Avoiding reduces your anxiety for a short while, so you end up avoiding more and more. Eventually, you are avoiding so much that your life ends up shrinking and you get dissatisfied with that.
> **Matthew:** But what if I tried eating solid food again, and it didn't work and I choked again?
> **Clinician:** That sounds like an important point. So how about if we looked at all the foods that you have cut out over time, and then we start working our way through the ones that you have never actually choked on?
> **Matthew:** So you mean something like starting with boiled potatoes, and then apples, and so on?
> **Clinician:** Well, let's start at the beginning and work out a list based on your experience of actual choking or fear of choking, going from the least risky to the scariest. So, if we start with boiled potatoes at the bottom of the "scary" list, what would be right at the top?
> **Matthew:** Beef, definitely—that is what I choked on at the start of all this. Okay, I will start that list. Can I do that for homework, because then I can ask my family to list the foods that I stopped eating, and when?
> **Clinician:** Sure. Make sure to rate how anxiety-provoking you think it would be to eat each food on your list. So, if beef is at the top of your list, what would you rate that on a scale of zero to 100?
> **Matthew:** One hundred—no doubt.
> **Clinician:** Okay, and what about nonsolid food?
> **Matthew:** Not anxiety-provoking at all...
> **Clinician:** So that would be a zero. And where would boiled potatoes be?

Matthew: Well, I never did choke on them. I just cut them out to be safe. So maybe a 25.

In this case, you want Matthew to start exposure by generating a hierarchy. Matthew is currently eating no solid food and finds even thinking about solid food anxiety-provoking. In making a hierarchy and thinking about very feared foods (e.g., beef), Matthew will start to engage in approaching feared stimuli (i.e., thoughts of eating feared foods) and reduce his avoidance. Thus, he is starting to engage in exposure at a low level, and his physician can use this to further engage him in exposure. Note that what Matthew's physician is *not* doing at this stage is committing to work very slowly through the hierarchy as the initial exposure.

Clinician: So, let's look at this hierarchy. I see you have a bunch of foods—boiled potatoes, solid ice cream, scrambled eggs, well-cooked pasta with sauce, bananas, and pancakes that are all around a 25 to 35.
Matthew: Yeah. I cut out all of those because it seemed like a good idea to just play it safe. But I was eating those before.
Clinician: So it seems like you are not very scared of eating those. Indeed, you ate them in the past after the choking episode and did just fine. So I am thinking we could introduce those foods back into your diet this week.
Matthew: All of them? What about just starting with ice cream? That seems like a safer way to go.
Clinician: Well, I think it is a question of whether or not you want to get on with your life. If we start with just one food, we are going to be working our way through this list for months and months. The "play it safe" approach has taken you to a very dysfunctional place. I think we need to experiment with a different approach, and you are telling me that none of these foods are terribly anxiety-provoking.
Matthew: Okay, I don't like the idea, but I guess I was feeling better when I was eating those soft foods. I guess I have to start somewhere.

SUMMARY

Patients with EDs experience substantial fear of food and eating. All clinicians who work with such patients will see the impact of those fears and have the opportunity to use exposure to address associated anxiety. The following points are particularly noteworthy:

- Specific foods need to be addressed using exposure. How they will be addressed will vary according to the nature of the fear associated with the food. In some cases, patients avoid foods to reduce the fear that they

will binge on them. In other cases, the foods are avoided secondary to the fear that eating some foods will result in uncontrollable weight gain.
- Fear of uncontrollable weight gain requires different uses of exposure, according to whether or not the patient is underweight and needs to gain weight as part of the treatment. While extremely low-weight patients may need to gain weight before starting exposure, some low-weight patients who are clearly engaging in voluntary treatment can use exposure to help them gain weight.
- Fears of specific foods or classes of food can be addressed using exposure, and this is a particularly useful approach when working with some manifestations of ARFID.

11

Cue Exposure for Binge Eating

As noted in the previous chapter, experiences of excessive eating that are commonly accompanied by a perceived loss of control over eating (i.e., binge eating) are important transdiagnostic phenomena in many individuals with EDs. Frequently, the development of binge eating occurs in response to prolonged dietary restraint. Thus, it is a process that is largely driven by biological processes activated via starvation, whether intentional or not (Fairburn & Harrison, 2003). It follows that one of the most important tools in decreasing binge eating is facilitating patients' resumption of normalized food intake (and weight regain if necessary), so that daily energy needs are consistently met. As demonstrated in Chapter 10, exposure can be used to facilitate this process and to decrease avoidance of feared foods and use of safety behaviors. However, many of your patients may continue to experience recurrent difficulties with binge-eating episodes despite establishing a more normalized diet, often without clear awareness of the underlying reasons for bingeing.

> Through repeated experience, Ruth learned that eating rich foods decreased her emotional distress. For instance, when upset as a young child, her family often attempted to comfort her via offering rich foods. Later in childhood, Ruth sought out these foods to reduce her stress around typical issues (e.g., academics, social relationships). Ruth was a larger-bodied child, who became quite self-conscious because of her size. She subsequently developed an ED, which was initially marked by significant dietary restraint that eventually gave way to persistent binge-eating episodes. Over time, Ruth noticed that the binge eating had a temporary calming effect on her, even though she found the binge eating very upsetting. The binge-eating episodes began to occur more frequently when she was experiencing negative moods—particularly in the evening hours when she became stressed while studying her school materials.
>
> With her family's support and encouragement, Ruth sought therapy for her ED. In the initial phase of her treatment, Ruth was successful in adhering to a structured dietary plan that included three well-balanced meals per day and snacks between the meals. Unfortunately, to the surprise of both Ruth

and her treatment providers, her binge-eating episodes continued despite no longer feeling the extreme hunger that had accompanied her dietary restraint. She continued to binge at nearly the same frequency that she had been prior to beginning therapy, and these episodes remained strongly associated with her experiences of negative emotions.

Ruth's case illustrates a relatively common occurrence among patients with binge-eating problems. The mere normalization of eating habits (and reintroduction of forbidden foods) does not produce the desired and expected reduction in bingeing episodes. This pattern can be particularly distressing because it is often associated with weight gain (as the binge episodes now happen on top of a normalized dietary intake). What might account for the continuation of overeating when one's energy needs are consistently being met? Here, it is important to consider the wider learning experience and the role of the cues that exist in the environment that might trigger eating behavior.[1]

THEORETICAL UNDERPINNINGS OF CUE EXPOSURE

The pioneering work of Jansen and colleagues (Jansen, 1998; Jansen, Broekmate, & Heymans, 1992; Jansen, Van den Hout, De Loof, Zandbergen, & Griez, 1989) has produced an empirically supported behavioral model of binge eating that is based on key principles of Pavlovian (i.e., classical) conditioning. You will likely recall hearing about Pavlovian conditioning in dogs and other animals, which learned to anticipate the arrival of food when presented with a neutral stimulus (e.g., the sound of a metronome). Although dogs require no experience or learning to salivate in response to being given food (i.e., an unconditional response), the food needed to be paired with the metronome sound repeatedly for the dogs to learn that the mere sound of the metronome signaled the imminent arrival of food (as evidenced by their salivation). Thus, a previously neutral stimulus that evoked no noteworthy response in dogs (the sound of a metronome) developed the "power" to elicit a strong physiological appetitive response via its repetitive pairing with the presentation of food.

Another way to think about this is to recognize that our (and dogs') bodies prefer to remain in a state of homeostasis. Food requires activation of digestive processes that normally return the body to homeostasis. When food is repeatedly consumed under predictable conditions (e.g., a time of day, in a particular location), our bodies initiate the digestive processes in anticipation of the food—in dogs, this can be observed via salivation—which helps us more effectively return

---

1. Cue exposure has been tested in relation to both prebinge cues and prepurge cues. However, given that research more strongly supports the impact of working with prebinge cues but not prepurge cues (Bulik, Sullivan, Carter, McIntosh, & Joyce, 1998), this chapter will focus on cue exposure for bingeing rather than purging.

to homeostasis after eating. However, if these processes are started and you break the normal pattern of eating, you will likely experience hunger or craving because your body is now prepared to digest food that has not actually been consumed. In fact, the anticipatory digestive processes have actually pulled you out of a homeostatic state, and the easiest way to return to that state is to eat—even if you have consumed sufficient food for the day.

The research of Jansen and others suggests that some of the recurrent binge-eating problems that many of your patients experience are similar to the recurrent salivary behaviors observed in Pavlov's dogs. Both are learned (i.e., conditioned) digestive responses to cues that were present when the responses were initially being provoked by actual food. Furthermore, both involve the initiation of digestive processes and physiological sensations that are experienced as an intense craving to consume food, which can often prove difficult to resist.

In many individuals who struggle with binge eating after resuming normal eating, binge-eating episodes are often elicited by contextual cues that were previously present prior to binge episodes. Common examples of these binge-eating cues include various forms of sensory experience with foods (e.g., seeing, touching, smelling, tasting), physical location and time of day when binges occurred, and any physiological sensations or negative emotional states preceding binge eating episodes (Bongers & Jansen, 2017). It should be noted that the stimuli that develop into binge-eating cues are often idiosyncratic and dependent on your patient's own set of experiences. To illustrate, Jansen et al. (1989) described a patient whose binge-eating cues included the style of clothing she typically wore and the magazines that she read during binge episodes.

A similar example is that of a male patient who described any "time to myself" as a cue for strong binge-eating cravings. Like many patients who recurrently binge, this patient was very ashamed of his bingeing and subsequently tried to do it only privately, which was challenging when living in an apartment with three roommates. He described experiencing an intense craving to binge whenever his roommates would all leave the apartment together.

Cue exposure works by targeting the conditioned physiological processes (i.e., initiation of digestive processes) and the subjective experience of these (i.e., cravings) that occur in relation to patients' typical binge cues. Here, it is again important to revisit some basics of Pavlovian conditioning. After dogs were conditioned to salivate in response to a previously neutral stimulus (metronome sound), they were then put through an *extinction learning* phase in which they were exposed to the sound of the metronome, which was not followed by the presentation of food. With enough repeated trials, the dogs learned that the metronome no longer predicted the arrival of food, and they stopped salivating as a result.

For humans as well as dogs, the essence of cue exposure is extinction learning. Your patients with binge-eating difficulties need to confront the typical stimuli that often cue their cravings to overeat, and this exposure must be paired with the prevention of binge eating. Doing so will yield similar effects to those observed in Pavlov's extinction learning—the cravings to binge will weaken over time with sufficient exposure. Put differently, your patients will learn that their typical binge-eating cues no longer predict overconsumption of food, and this new learning will inhibit the previous association between the environmental cues and binge-eating behaviors (Jansen, Schyns, Bongers, & van den Akker, 2016). As with fear learning, it is important to remember that the initial learning never goes away. Moreover, extinction learning (or inhibitory learning) is often weaker than the original learning. So it can spontaneously reappear. You will want to warn your patients about this, so that they can re-engage with exposure to strengthen the inhibitory learning.

NOTABLE DIFFERENCES FROM TRADITIONAL EXPOSURE

Most of the other forms of exposure therapy described in this book involve encouraging patients to confront stimuli that evoke fear. Whether it be calorically dense foods, mirrors, bathing suits, choking sensations, or standing on a scale, the predominant emotional response to these stimuli among most ED patients is fear. A majority of ED patients respond to their fear of these stimuli by attempting to avoid them and/or using safety behaviors to neutralize perceived threat. It follows that exposure therapy to address these issues takes the form of patients confronting their feared stimuli and not engaging in any safety behaviors.

Cue exposure to address binge eating has some notable differences from these other forms of "traditional" exposure therapy for EDs. First, rather than fear, individuals with binge-eating difficulties are likely to experience other emotional and physiological responses to cue exposure. These experiences include strong physiological cravings to consume food as well as positive expectancies related to the anticipation of consuming rich, palatable foods and subsequent disappointment when these cravings are not fulfilled. Given binge-eating patients' positive expectancies regarding food consumption, there is less of a tendency to engage in avoidance or safety behaviors. Rather, the primary behavioral response that you need to discourage in cue exposure is your patients actually binge eating. If binge eating continues to follow exposure to conditioned cues to binge, then your patient will not experience sufficient learning to inhibit their association between these cues and the consequent binge episodes.

IMPLEMENTING CUE EXPOSURE

Because cue exposure does not instinctively make sense to many people, implementing cue exposure can require even more psychoeducation and preparatory work (e.g., identifying cues) than other forms of exposure, as will be explained in the following discussion. Without due attention to that work, the implementation is unlikely to be successful.

Educating Your Patient

As noted in Chapter 7, providing your patients with psychoeducation about the maintenance of their ED and the rationale for exposure therapy is a crucial step in ensuring their investment and cooperation in carrying out treatment. Given some of the differences in the theoretical underpinnings and core objectives of cue exposure as compared to other forms of exposure, you will likely need to provide some specialized education prior to staring cue exposure.

In our experience, cue exposure is not as intuitive to patients as other forms of exposure. Whereas many patients have little difficulty grasping the rationale to "face their fears," the idea of confronting things that are associated with their bingeing behaviors is not understood as easily. This may be due partly to patients receiving advice from family, friends, healthcare professionals, or even 12-step-based support groups that foods and other cues that are associated with the individual's bingeing *should* be avoided. As such, your education about the maintenance of binge eating and cue exposure treatment rationale may fly in the face of what your patient has come to believe is the best way to manage their problem and/or might strike them as counterintuitive (e.g., "You want me to just *sit* in front of food, when you know that the food makes me want to eat it?").

Psychoeducation for your patient should include conveying an understanding that binge eating can often continue even after successful resumption of appropriate dietary intake. This information alone is often very relieving to patients, who can be extremely frustrated with themselves due to a perceived lack of willpower or characterological flaw. Education should also emphasize the role of stimuli that have become conditioned cues for strong eating cravings and binge behaviors by virtue of their previous pairing with bingeing episodes. Providing a rationale for cue exposure should include a description of extinction learning principles and how they will apply to your patient's idiosyncratic binge cues. This will aid in creating an expectation of benefit in your patient at the outset of cue exposure.

> **Devin:** I'm really frustrated that I keep on bingeing. I don't know why it keeps happening because I've done a good job with sticking to the eating plan.
> **Clinician:** I can understand your frustration, and I'm glad that you've done well with normalizing your eating. It might surprise you to learn that this can happen for a lot of people who are trying to stop their bingeing. It unfortunately persists even after you are no longer withholding food from yourself.
> **Devin:** You're saying a lot of people have this experience?
> **Clinician:** Yes.
> **Devin:** Well, I guess I feel a little better knowing that I'm not the only one. Any idea why this keeps happening to me? I really want to cut it out. It only feels good for a bit before I just get really guilty.

Clinician: Based on what you've described in some of our previous meetings, I think the bingeing keeps happening because you continue to encounter things that you've come to associate with your binges. In other words, there were likely some consistent things you came across or experiences that you had before you binged, and these things now act as "cues" for your bingeing because they probably make you crave the food when you run into them.

Devin: That sounds a little like my cat. She always runs over to her food bowl and meows when she hears me coming down the stairs in the morning. She didn't do that before, but it seems like she knows I'm going to feed her as soon as she hears my footsteps on the stairs.

Clinician: Exactly! Your cat has learned to expect she'll be fed when she hears you on the stairs. I'm guessing just the sound of this makes her crave the food and she gets excited. This is similar to your issue with bingeing. You have likely learned to expect that certain things, whether it be foods, places, or even your own feelings, are associated with bingeing, and these things increase your cravings.

Devin: That makes sense. One thing I've definitely noticed is that when I sit in my comfy recliner and watch *The Big Bang Theory*, I wind up bingeing on cookies pretty often. It sometimes happens to me even though it's right after dinner and I'm not even a bit hungry.

Clinician: It sounds to me like your comfy recliner and *The Big Bang Theory* were things that were often associated with your past bingeing, and they developed the ability to make you crave food. Now when you sit in the recliner and watch the show, you get cravings that are hard to ignore.

Devin: Yeah, I think you're right. Before I even go sit down or turn on the TV, I'm not even thinking about the cookies. But as soon as I do it, it's like I'm reminded of how good the cookies would taste.

Note that drawing parallels to the ways in which animals behave under conditions when they have come to expect food (e.g., Devin's cat) often helps patients grasp the concepts underpinning cue exposure.

Identifying Appropriate Cues

In the previous example, Devin appeared to have some knowledge of the stimuli (i.e., cues) that evoked strong binge-eating cravings. In this situation, the clinician can simply proceed with asking questions to identify further stimuli that act as cues to binge. This can be done in the format of a functional assessment of the binge-eating behaviors and related symptoms (see Chapter 6).

However, it is important to note that many of your patients may not be able to identify the full range of their binge-eating cues. Because the stimuli that cue many patients' binges are multifaceted, your patients may be able to report some aspects of a given stimulus or cue scenario but might fail to recognize other aspects. To illustrate, a patient may appropriately recognize that being in close proximity to donuts is a cue for his binge eating, while failing to recognize that feeling boredom when in the presence of the donuts is an equally powerful cue for his bingeing.

Other patients may genuinely appear to lack all knowledge of the antecedent cues to their bingeing episodes. Accordingly, when helping your patients identify their binge cues, it is important that you ask follow-up questions and, when warranted, encourage your patient to engage in careful self-monitoring of various cues that they notice preceding their binge-eating urges and/or behaviors. This self-monitoring should include specific information about the context in which the binge urges/behaviors occurred, such as the physical location and time of day, as well as the thoughts, emotions, and physical sensations that your patient was experiencing. The monitoring form provided in Figure 11.1 is an example of a tool that patients can use in their self-monitoring. A blank version of the form is included in the appendix.

Instructions:
Please use this form to record as much information as you can whenever you notice an increased urge to binge or after you have binged.

Day & time	Where were you? What was going on around you?	What body sensations were you experiencing?	What thoughts were you having?	What emotions were you feeling?
Tuesday 8:30pm	I was in my kitchen at home. I had just finished cleaning up from supper, when my sister called me. We wound up getting into an argument over how we're going to take care of my father after his surgery.	A lot of tension in my neck and shoulders. I was hot and a little bit sweaty.	"Why does she always have to belittle me?" "I wish she hadn't called in the first place!"	Anger, frustration

Figure 11.1. Binge cue monitoring form.

Conducting Cue Exposure

Once you have identified the stimuli that cue your patient's binge eating, you can begin the process of exposure to these cues. As discussed in Chapter 9, you have the option of creating a hierarchy with your patient in which you would collaborate to arrange the cue stimuli in order from the lowest to the highest anticipated intensity of cravings. As an alternative to creating a hierarchy, you can simply ask your patient to choose a cue that they believe will be challenging, yet manageable for them to confront without engaging in any subsequent binge behaviors.

During cue exposure, patients are instructed to engage with the cue stimuli and attend closely to the cravings that are evoked (vs. attempting to avoid or suppress cravings). In the context of food-related interactions, you can encourage your patient to engage with the food in a variety of ways, including touching, smelling, and tasting the food. Different forms of these food interactions can be "mixed and matched" to titrate binge cravings to an appropriate level.

> **Clinician:** We've been holding the box of chocolates for a few minutes now. Tell me where your cravings are at.
>
> **Gary:** They're actually not too high. I really don't have much of an urge to binge right now.
>
> **Clinician:** Okay, it sounds like we're ready to go a step further. How about you open the box and take a good whiff of the chocolate?
>
> **Gary:** Um, okay (*opens box and smells*). Mmmm, I love that smell (*smells again*). They smell so good. And they look really good, too.
>
> **Clinician:** Do you notice any change in your cravings right now, Gary?
>
> **Gary:** Oh, yeah, absolutely. I'm really feeling strong cravings now after I opened the box and smelled them.
>
> **Clinician:** Can you describe that feeling a little bit more?
>
> **Gary:** Well, it's hard to describe. I just really feel like I want to eat all this chocolate right now. It kind of feels similar to being excited about something good that'll happen. I feel it most in my stomach.
>
> **Clinician:** Okay, good. Let's continue to have you hold the box and smell chocolate every so often. If you'd like, try taking out a few of the chocolates and holding them. Keep paying attention to your cravings and allowing yourself to feel them.

IMPORTANT CONSIDERATIONS

Cue exposure should be considered and implemented in context. You should think about when it is appropriate to begin such exposure, your own impact on the learning process, and where and under what conditions cue exposure should be conducted.

When to Begin

Although there are few contraindications to beginning cue exposure as soon as possible within a course of treatment, you need to assess your patient's dietary habits outside of his binges. If your assessment reveals consistent patterns of dietary restraint, you should consider delaying cue exposure temporarily while you encourage your patient to establish improved nutritional stability, in which his energy needs are consistently met. The purpose of this is to mitigate the biological contributors to his binge eating that are fueled by the ongoing efforts to withhold food. Not doing so runs the risk of your patient being "set up" to binge, which, of course, will only further strengthen the association between his binge cues and binge eating behavior. In summary, you want to use nutritional stabilization as your primary strategy to reduce binge eating to the degree possible and then use cue exposure as potential secondary strategy to address residual binge eating.

The Clinician as a Safety Signal

Your mere presence in the room when your patient is engaging in cue exposure could unintentionally preclude your patient from maximizing the inhibitory learning that takes place during exposure. This is because your patient may not experience as intense of food cravings as she typically does, due to your presence. Bear in mind that you were not present during any of her previous binges. Thus, you are a new stimulus in the binge eating context, and you are a stimulus that she does not associate with bingeing. We have heard from many patients undergoing cue exposure that the presence of a clinician has the effect of artificially suppressing cravings. Fortunately, Jansen et al. (1992) have outlined a useful strategy that allows for your presence to be progressively "faded" from the cue exposure context. Following this strategy, you would first conduct cue exposure while being present in the room with your patient before removing yourself from the room at a later time, placing yourself in an adjacent office so that you are still on hand to assist your patient as needed. Finally, you can plan with your patient ahead of time that your only involvement in a subsequent cue exposure session will be via phone.

Conducting Exposure in the Binge-Eating Context

Just as your presence was not a component of your patient's previous bingeing episodes, her binge eating also very likely did not occur in your clinical workplace. Because of the importance of trying to replicate your patient's previous binge-eating context and cues as much as possible (Jansen, Schyns, et al., 2016), it is important that you make efforts to facilitate cue exposure in the actual context(s) in which your patient's prior bingeing occurred. In addition to strongly encouraging your patient to complete cue exposure homework exercises at home, you may consider conducting at least some of your cue exposure sessions with your patient in the necessary context (e.g., at a crowded food court in a mall, using the drive-thru window at a fast food restaurant, etc.). As we have discussed with other forms of exposure, the treatment tends to work best when it is conducted in settings and under situational conditions that are uniquely pertinent to your patients.

SUMMARY

Many of your patients who have experienced difficulties with binge eating will likely continue to do so even after nutritional stabilization because a variety of cues they encounter elicit strong food cravings. Cue exposure is a helpful technique to address binge eating. It involves confronting the cues that typically elicit heightened food cue reactivity (i.e., cravings), while preventing the subsequent response of bingeing. In this process, your patients will experience inhibitory learning, in which they will come to learn that their binge cues are no longer predictive of an actual episode of binge eating. This will have the effect of substantially weakening cravings that occur in association with exposure to binge eating cues.

12

Weighing and Weight Exposure

In almost every evidence-based therapy for EDs, weighing your patient openly (i.e., with your patient seeing and discussing their weight) is an integral part of treatment (Waller & Mountford, 2015). Despite this, a very substantial number of clinicians actively or passively avoid weighing their patients in this way (e.g., Forbush, Richardson, & Bohrer, 2015; Mulkens, de Vos, de Graaff, & Waller, 2018; Waller, Stringer, & Meyer, 2012). Some report that they blind weigh their patients (so that patients are weighed but do not know their weight), some pass on the responsibility to others, and some work on the assumption that they can tell if their patients change weight "by eye." None of these approaches will meet your patients' need to learn that food is not their enemy. Indeed, by joining in with your patients (or even leading your patients) in avoiding knowing their weight, you are likely to enhance your patients' concerns about their weight.

WHY WEIGH YOUR PATIENTS?

Waller and Mountford (2015) detail the reasons for weighing all patients with EDs. To start, you need to ensure your patient's safety and identify changes in eating patterns when food diaries are unreliable. You also want to teach safety and tolerance of the process of being weighed (including learning that weight does not change if one does not check or avoid one's body), which will ultimately reduce associated anxiety. Ultimately, you want your patient to realize that their weight is just one piece of data about their body—one that does not need to be so emotionally laden. Finally, you will use weighing to modify the "broken cognitive link" between eating and weight gain. Although exposure is commonly associated with behavioral and cognitive-behavioral therapy (CBT) approaches, Waller and Mountford (2015) stress that such weighing is recommended as a core element in most evidence-based therapies for EDs. Therefore, understanding the impact of weighing exposure on eating pathology extends beyond behavioral and CBT approaches to EDs.

ADDRESSING YOUR OWN ANXIETY ABOUT WEIGHT AND WEIGHING

All of your ED patients should be weighed openly, particularly if you are using an evidence-based therapy such as CBT-ED or family-based therapy (Waller & Mountford, 2015). So that really just leaves you with the question of when to do so. The answer to that question is quite simple: you should weigh your patients at every session. Unfortunately, as previously noted, clinical practice frequently deviates from evidence-based approaches (e.g., Mulkens et al., 2018; Tobin, Banker, Weisberg, & Bowers, 2007; Waller et al., 2012), so this may not currently be part of your routine practice. If you are new to weighing your patient at every session, there are several considerations you will want to keep in mind.

First, it is important to realize that while your patients will undoubtedly be anxious about their weight, relatively few patients are so anxious about the weighing process that they adamantly refuse to be weighed. However, if one of your patients does refuse, you will need to address this straight away. In short, you will need to use exposure to overcome your patient's avoidance of awareness of her weight. To do this, you also may need to overcome your own concerns about weighing your patients.

Three common factors appear to drive clinician reluctance to weigh patients. One is *our concern that our patients will be unduly distressed* by knowing their weight. Certainly, many patients will try to convey that weighing is simply too distressing to tolerate; this is often manifested via statements like the following:

- "But if you weigh me, I will have to starve myself."
- "If I know my weight, then I will just end up bingeing."
- "I can't do therapy if it means being weighed."
- "None of my other therapists have ever wanted to weigh me."

When your patients say things like this, they are trying to reduce the likelihood that you will follow through with weighing. If you give in, they will have succeeded in engaging you as an active participant in their avoidance. Often, these statements represent a reinforced behavior, in that they have helped patients to successfully avoid being weighed by previous clinicians. Despite this, many of these same patients will agree to be weighed when weighing is presented in a matter-of-fact way. However, a few (particularly those whose behavior has been reinforced by multiple clinicians) may try this behavior several times to avoid weighing because it has been so successful in the past. With such patients, you will have to persevere to extinguish this reinforced behavior. If necessary, we find it important to stress that we cannot offer therapy if our patients are not willing to be weighed (note that we have not had any patients decline at this point). Protesting weighing also may spontaneously re-emerge in some highly reinforced patients, particularly if other aspects of treatment or life are anxiety-provoking. Don't get caught off guard or acquiesce. If you give in, you will put your patient on an intermittent schedule of reinforcement, and weighing will become that much more difficult. If you are committed to and consistent with weighing, in contrast, it will become routine, straightforward, and, ultimately, even a little boring (which, you will remember from earlier, is a positive stage in treating anxiety).

The second factor that makes us less likely to weigh patients is *our own characteristics as clinicians*. For instance, we are less likely to use exposure-based methods (including weighing) as we get older and if we are more anxious as individuals (Turner, Tatham, Lant, Mountford, & Waller, 2014). Mulkens et al. (2018) also have shown that we are less likely to weigh patients if we emphasize the clinical utility of developing the therapeutic relationship. Although the desire to build a strong therapeutic relationship is understandable, you cannot let such a desire interfere with the implementation of core elements of treatment that are likely to benefit your patients. As we will note repeatedly in this book, when working with ED patients, you must keep in mind Wilson, Fairburn, & Agras's (1997) recommendation that the most effective therapeutic relationship in working with EDs is one that is based on balancing empathy with firmness. Just as an oncologist cannot remove unpleasant elements of treatment (e.g., chemotherapy and radiation) secondary to a desire to be liked, you cannot avoid weighing. Finally, our own anxiety about weighing patients is something that we should address through mechanisms such as exposure for exposure therapists (Farrell, Deacon, Dixon, & Lickel, 2013), rather than allowing our own concerns to divert us from delivering components of treatment that will be beneficial for our patients. As noted in Chapter 9, you should be teaching your patients to view exposure as a lifestyle. You need to "walk the walk" and similarly embrace a lifestyle in which you approach, not avoid, the situations that cause you anxiety.

The third and final factor that can reduce our likelihood of weighing patients appropriately (or at all) is *service configuration and philosophy*. Some services are configured in ways that emphasize professional boundaries (e.g., "The dietitian weighs patients, and the therapist does the CBT, and they should not overlap, in case one of them looks unnecessary, or they argue over who does what"). However, that argument is not clinically justified (see Chapter 18 for more in-depth discussion). Indeed, in many cases, other services are effectively risk-avoidant and will treat the risk of a few patients being distressed as more important than the likelihood of helping a much larger number of patients. An example of this risk avoidance can be seen in this exchange between a newly employed clinician and her supervisor:

> **Supervisor:** Welcome aboard. Now, you have worked in an eating disorder treatment center previously, so let's just check on what you usually do from the first session. I just want to make sure that you are on track. . . . To start, one of the things that I want to check on is how you weigh your patients each time you see them.
> **Clinician:** Well, in my last job, we were told to suggest it to our patients—to say that it might be a good idea to weigh them, and to see if they were okay with that. If a patient wasn't okay with weighing, then we waited to

see if they would agree to be weighed later in therapy. Or if we thought they wouldn't be okay with being weighed, that we might chase them out of treatment, then we didn't ask and waited to see if they would come around to it.

Supervisor: Was there a particular reason for that approach?

Clinician: Not really—just that we did not want to chase our patients away. Patients are so ambivalent—it just feels really easy to lose them.

Supervisor: So did that work? Did patients stay in therapy more because of this strategy? Did you manage to get them weighed in time?

Clinician: I don't really know if they stayed in therapy more. Hard to know really, but we assumed it worked. I know that if we pushed the patients to be weighed later because we were worried about them, they got really anxious and that was when they dropped out. Sometimes they would let us weigh them if we promised not to tell them what they weighed.

Supervisor: Right. Well, here we all weigh all of our patients openly at every session, so that is something that we are going to have to get you doing from the beginning. That is going to make you at least a little anxious, I suspect.

Clinician: Afraid so. What if they refuse, or they don't come back?

Supervisor: That sounds like you are trying to rationalize avoidance to reduce your own anxiety. Let's give it a try, cope with your fear, and we will see if you get less anxious as you get used to weighing them.

Six months later, at a routine review of the therapist's progress in the job, the following exchange took place. It reflects the degree to which the therapist had overcome her anxiety about weighing patients, and had learned from her contrasting experiences:

Supervisor: Way back when you started, I told you that you would need to weigh all of your patients openly. You were worried about that, but I told you that you should go ahead. Now, since then I know that you have been weighing them openly, so how is your anxiety about doing so?

Clinician: It seems ridiculous to me now that I was worried about weighing them, though I really was and I sort of hated you for telling me to do it. But I have been weighing in every first session, and nearly every patient has been fine with it. In the couple of cases where my patient has said, "Do I have to?" or "It will make me restrict," I have been firm. No one has run off, and the strangest thing is that they seem to just accept it in subsequent sessions, even if they don't like it.

Supervisor: So what have you learned?

Clinician: I think that the first thing that I have learned is that patients are not as fragile as I thought they were. The other thing, though, is that I have learned that how we ask the question really matters. In my last job, we would say to the patient that "it might be a good idea if I were to weigh you," and about half said, "No thanks." In fact, we were so worried that even asking the patient might upset them that we very often did not even ask, and we assumed that the patient would not be happy to be weighed. In *this* job, I tell the patient that "it is time to weigh you"—very matter of fact, and almost everyone is absolutely fine with it, and the others agree when I explain why.

Supervisor: So how is your anxiety regarding weighing?

Clinician: Gone. It's just part of the therapy, and it works. I remember you talking about exposure therapy for the therapist, and it feels like that had worked on me within about 2 weeks. Now, I get my trainees to do the same thing, and I see it in action—their fear just fades, and fast. They also learn you shouldn't avoid clinical tasks that make you anxious. You can handle it. In my last job, I reckon that I probably ended up weighing about half of my patients, but here it is 100%.

In conclusion, you should weigh your patient at each session and ensure that they have processed this (seeing the weight at the time; charting the weight jointly). That means that we need to overcome any reluctance on the part of the patient, any beliefs or anxieties that we hold, and service-level obstructions.

USING EXPOSURE TO ADDRESS YOUR PATIENTS ANXIETY ABOUT WEIGHT AND WEIGHING

There are a number of complementary exposure strategies that you can use to reduce your patients' anxiety about weighing. It is likely that you already use at least some of these. However, you also might need to consider the ways in which you avoid these strategies (and consider ways to overcome that avoidance). These exposure strategies include the following:

- Starting to talk about weight at the assessment session and from the beginning of therapy itself;
- Talking about weight freely and in a matter-of-fact way;
- Making sure that weighing scales are plainly visible in the room throughout the session;
- Keeping the patient's weight chart visible on the desk; and
- Creating weight charts that demonstrate the full range of weight that an underweight patient needs to gain.

In our experience, many clinicians avoid some or all of these, for fear of distressing their ED patients. This avoidance usually results in later difficulties in therapy (e.g., the need to get the scales out, making weighing more of an "event";

having to revise the apparent targets on the weight chart when the patient gains more than is shown).

It is important to remember, however, that these are relatively low-level ways of beginning exposure to weighing when you consider the anxiety that likely will be evoked when you actually weigh your patients. Greater anxiety will often be driven by your patients' concerns about what they will weigh. Yet, to maximize the benefit of exposure in the form of weighing, you will often need to strategically and purposefully *increase* weighing anxiety.

Weighing exposure can be viewed as successful when your patient experiences increased tolerance to weighing over multiple weighing experiences. This will typically be accompanied by a reduction in fear. Consistent with previous chapters, when conducting weighing exposure, we recommend that you aim for anxiety to be as high as your patient can tolerate at the point of weighing, so that the learning can be rapidly maximized. Therefore, you should optimally weigh your patients *after* you have discussed what they have eaten and its potential consequences in enough detail to activate the "hot" cognitions that underpin elevated emotional experiences (see Waller & Mountford, 2015, for additional discussion of weighing patients).

In the following example, note that the therapist adheres to principles of the inhibitory learning approach. He deliberately does not weigh Zara immediately once she has made her weight prediction but instead maintains the focus on feared experiences (the "roll of fat"; other people's perceptions) and even accentuates them by getting her to point to the perceived roll of fat. The therapist also does not extend the period of exposure to weighing with the aim of seeking within-session anxiety reduction. Instead the focus is (a) on violating the harm expectancy of 3-kilogram weight gain with normalized eating and (b) then to repeat that experience the following week since Zara is clearly doubtful and needs more inhibitory learning.

> **Clinician:** Right, we have your diary here, and it looks as though you have eaten pretty much everything that we planned for you over the week. You missed a couple of snacks, but you didn't binge or vomit. So that means that you have had about 2,000 calories per day, you have eaten the planned foods that you were scared of, including the biscuits, and you have kept it down. Well done! How does that sound to you?
>
> **Zara:** Horrible. I hadn't looked at it like that before. That is such a lot of food.
>
> **Clinician:** So what do you think will have happened to your weight? Last week, you predicted that eating this way would make you gain at least a kilo, but you sounded less worried then. What is your prediction now that you have eaten all that?
>
> **Zara:** Far more than that—I can feel it as we talk about it. It must be 2 kilos or even a bit more—it can't be less than that.
>
> **Clinician:** Tell me more about the feeling.

Zara: It's like a roll of fat on my belly. I'm not sure how to explain it. The feeling is really revolting. I am sure that you must be able to see it.
Clinician: Show me where you mean.
Zara: Sort of here (*points to her navel and round to her back*).
Clinician: Does it feel hard? Soft? Firm? Wobbly?
Zara: I hate talking about this—I think everyone will see the fat and how much weight I have gained.
Clinician: You expect people to comment on it?
Zara: Of course, they will. And I think it must be nearer to 3 kilos. Not just 2.
Clinician: So let's find out. How anxious are you feeling right now, on that zero-to-100 scale?
Zara: At least 100.
Therapist: Okay, well, we can see if that is the same in coming weeks (*weighs Zara*).
Clinician: So, your weight has stayed almost exactly the same—up by just 100 grams.
Zara: I just don't think that is right. How on earth can that be right?
Clinician: Then you will need to find out if eating the same amount next time has the effect that it felt like this week. Only let's introduce some new feared foods to go along with the ones you started eating this past week.

In summary, the goal is to repeat this experience over multiple weeks to determine whether Zara's weight gain predictions come true or not and to mix up the context by adding new foods. Typically, anxiety will fall when the weight gain predictions do not come true. In some cases, however, your patients will gain weight (especially if weight gain is a target of therapy because your patient is underweight). Then the focus will be on learning to tolerate that weight gain. Body image exposure (see Chapter 13) can be particularly helpful in accomplishing this.

Safety Behaviors Associated With Weighing

There are a number of anxiety reduction methods that patients routinely use around the experience of weighing. You need to be aware of these behaviors, so that you can address them when your patients want to use them and you are tempted to let them. This involves two steps. First, you need to make it clear to your patients that they want to use these behaviors to reduce their anxiety. By making the anxiety-reduction function of the behaviors overt, you make it harder for your patient to represent those behaviors as reasonable actions; you also make a direct connection to psychoeducation for exposure so that you remind your patients of the rationale for resisting. Second, you have to help your patient actually resist the urge to engage in the safety behaviors. The aim here is to keep your patients' anxiety high enough for appropriate learning. Such safety behaviors include the following.

- *Allowing your patient to preweigh herself before coming to therapy.* Zara should be told that weighing herself at all between or before sessions is not helpful and should be avoided completely. This approach commonly means asking Zara to dispose of her own scales or store them where she cannot access them. The rationale is that we do not want Zara to be aware of her weight before the session, so that (a) she experiences the anxiety of not knowing her weight all week (for many patients, this anxiety will decrease naturally over that time); (b) she experiences the full anxiety associated with the process of being weighed by someone else after discussing eating to heighten "hot" cognitions (see the previous discussion) and clearly articulate the fear expectancy; and (c) she learns that her acute anxiety either falls or becomes more tolerable from session to session.
- *Weighing your patient as soon as she arrives in the clinic.* Patients will often ask if they can be weighed immediately after they arrive. Sometimes, a patient like Zara will ask you if she can jump straight onto the scales. Other times, before she even comes in to see you, she will ask the reception team or another staff member if they can weigh her or let her use the clinic scales. These are all safety behaviors. Zara is trying to alter the nature of the process of being weighed to reduce her anxiety as compared to being weighed when she is in the therapy room with you. You need to ensure that no team member (yourself included) allows her to use such safety behaviors.
- *Increasing the predictability of weighing.* Patients such as Zara will often try to ensure that weighing in the clinic is as predictable a process as possible by always wearing the same clothes, asking to always be weighed on the same set of scales, making sure the scales are always placed in exactly the same place on the floor, always scheduling her appointment at the same time of day, etc. To maximize inhibitory learning, you need to ensure that this level of predictability is minimized. This can mean deliberately asking Zara to dress differently each week, moving the scales to different positions, using different sets of scales (calibrated to each other, without Zara knowing that), varying appointment times, and so on.

SUMMARY

Regular, open weighing is a critical component of evidence-based treatments for EDs. Weight provides critical information for violating patients' harm expectancies, and weighing offers a powerful learning opportunity for coping with anxiety. Although many clinicians collude with their patients in avoiding open weighing, your job is to tolerate your own anxiety about things such as patient dropout, while asking your patients to do likewise with their anxiety about knowing their weight. That means that we have to learn the same thing as the patient. However anxious we are when weighing our patients, we cannot be effective if we respond to our own anxiety by reducing the demands of the situation and cave on the critically important task of weighing our patients in an open and forthright manner.

# 13

Body Image Exposure

Body image disturbance plays a key role in the development, maintenance, and relapse processes for many ED patients. You are likely familiar with many of your patients attempting (in vain) to manage their negative body image by engaging in avoidance, comparison, and/or checking (i.e., safety) behaviors. Addressing your patients' negative body image will be critical when it presents as a maintaining component of an ED.

> Talia, whose immediate family all lived in higher weight bodies, had an 8-year history of atypical AN and a lifetime history of subclinical dietary restriction. Talia reported being a "a very chubby kid" who always wanted to be "normal." At the start of treatment, Talia was severely restricting her intake to less than 500 calories per day and experienced very irregular menses. Talia's clinical ED had started after she experimented with an 800 calorie per day diet at the suggestion of a physician friend. After she started losing weight, Talia gradually increased her restriction and ultimately was able to reach a target BMI of 26, which made her feel "normal though not skinny."
>
> With the help of her therapist, Talia successfully reinstated regular eating and increased her daily intake. During this time, she also gained approximately 27 pounds and reached a BMI of 30.5. The weight gain returned her to pre-ED weight and, in the words of her mother, her "family's traditional full-figured shape." Although Talia reported being happy with her progress in changing her eating and her increased energy, she remained "miserable" with the way her body looked and felt.
>
> Talia reported that whenever she sat, she tried to "sit lightly and perch" by constricting her buttocks and her thighs to limit how much her thighs spread. She also alternately avoided mirrors and used them to check if certain clothes helped to slim her. During the weekend, she would wear very baggy clothing so she could avoid thinking about her body. Talia refused to go to work or any social event without wearing body-shaping undergarments, even though she reported finding them very uncomfortable.
>
> Talia had given up going to the gym since gaining weight—reporting that "no one wants to see a whale like me lumbering around the gym." She also

> increasingly isolated herself socially, secondary to fear of getting comments about either her weight gain or what she was eating. Many of her long-standing friends had praised her for her weight loss and her self-control during the course of her ED.

Body image concerns typically are addressed after eating behaviors are stabilized (Fairburn, 2008; Trottier, Carter, MacDonald, McFarlane, & Olmsted, 2015). One advantage of this approach is that it provides time for patients who are going to gain weight to actually gain that weight and, at least partially, restore their weight. Teaching patients to tolerate or even appreciate their bodies when weight is significantly suppressed can be, in many ways, a waste of time since patients typically will have to relearn to tolerate their bodies at higher weights. At the same time, you do not need to wait until low-weight patients have completely reached their target weight. Once your patient is approaching a target weight, you can begin body image exposure work.

Exposure therapy for body image concerns is relevant to ED patients regardless of diagnosis. While it is commonly discussed in relation to patients who have regained weight or who are at a "normal" weight, it applies equally to those who have higher weight bodies. Patients like Talia, who live in higher-weight, stigmatized bodies, also must learn to tolerate their bodies in a social environment that encourages active disparagement of their bodies. These patients will often have their harm expectancies confirmed; as such, the goal will be to alter their ability to tolerate anxiety and negative emotions that accompany those experiences. For these patients, body image exposure may look something like exposure for social anxiety disorder, which frequently involves exposing patients to actual negative evaluation to enhance tolerance of such evaluation. You also may need to supplement exposure with assertiveness training.

MIRROR EXPOSURE

As noted in Chapter 5, the most studied form of body image exposure for EDs is mirror exposure. The term *mirror exposure* actually encompasses several related techniques, which means you have options in how to conduct mirror exposure. Despite some differences in how mirror exposure can be implemented, what each of the various forms of mirror exposure (see the following discussion) share in common is an emphasis on having patients view their bodies in a mirror while wearing "revealing" clothing with the aim of improving acceptance and tolerance of their physique. Please note that "revealing" in this setting should be appropriate to the context and simply means that your patients should be able to view their body shape rather than concealing it—so a leotard might be suitable in some cases, whereas casual clothes would be more suitable in others. This point is addressed further in the following discussion.

"Pure" Mirror Exposure

As an example of one particular form of mirror exposure, Talia could complete mirror exposure using the classic habituation paradigm. This approach is sometimes referred to as "pure" mirror exposure (Moreno-Dominguez, Rodriguez-Ruiz, Santaella, Jansen, & Tuschen-Caffier, 2012).

> **Clinician:** Thank you for wearing your swimsuit under your clothing today.
> **Talia:** I really didn't want to. I actually had to buy a new one. I bought it online because I couldn't stand the idea of actually trying on multiple suits in a store. Am I really going to have to look at myself wearing it? I've tried it on to make sure it fit, but haven't looked at myself in it.
> **Clinician:** So, as we discussed previously, exposure doesn't only help you change your eating behaviors. It can also change how you feel about your body.
> **Talia:** I don't think anything can change that. I hate looking this way. I wish I could eat the way I am eating now and still be thinner, like I was before. It's not fair—I'm not asking to be a supermodel—I just want to look like other normal women and be able to buy regular clothes without searching for plus sizes or shopping in a special store just for fat people.
> **Clinician:** I totally understand why you preferred a lower weight given all of the societal pressure. As we discussed, however, a key component of therapy is learning to live with whatever body you end up with when you are eating in a healthy manner; we can't change your genetics. Now, I am sure we could spend the rest of session discussing this and the fact that we live in a world that really does stigmatize people whose bodies are naturally bigger, but then we wouldn't have time for exposure. And this would just make it that much harder for us to do this next week because we would have avoided it this week. So let's go over to the mirror like we planned with you just wearing your swimsuit. I'll meet you over there. (*Talia takes off outer clothing and walks to mirror. She turns her body to the side and tearfully peeks at herself in mirror.*)
> **Clinician:** Okay. Now please walk up to the mirror so you are facing it and can see your whole body. About 4 to 5 feet from the mirror. Great. Now look at your body and pay attention to your feelings and thoughts. Please don't try to reduce your anxiety or discomfort while looking at your body. Stay focused on your body and feel your anxiety and discomfort. So what are you thinking and feeling as you look at your body?
> **Talia:** I feel so fat and gross. I can't stand to look at myself. No one can love me at this weight. I can't love me. I hate the way my stomach and legs look. And my boobs are so big again. Ugh . . .
> **Clinician:** On a scale of zero to 100, how much distress about your body are you experiencing?
> **Talia:** 95

Clinician: (*35 minutes later*) On that zero-to-100 scale, where are now?
Talia: It's hard to say. I still hate what I am seeing, but I feel somewhat calmer. Maybe resigned is a better word. I don't know . . . maybe 70.
Clinician: Okay. What have you learned from this first round of mirror exposure?
Talia: Hmmm. Hard to say . . . Actually, I don't think I realized it, but I think I thought that looking at my body would just make things worse and worse. I know it sounds crazy, but I sort feared I would just look fatter and fatter. Now I sort of just see my body. Don't get me wrong. I still don't like it, and I am not excited to do the homework I think you are about to give me. But I don't feel as badly as I did when we started.

Guided Mirror Exposure

Alternatively, Talia could be guided through exposure using a nonjudgmental approach during which the therapist would ask Talia to describe specific body parts as objectively as possible ("What do your legs look like?"). The therapist could then correct Talia if she moved into a judgmental stance.

Talia: My legs are hideous . . .
Clinician: Calling your legs hideous describes your reaction to your legs. Please describe your legs as objectively as possible. Imagine you were asking an artist to draw your legs. Hideous wouldn't tell the artist the shape or size or length of your legs. The artist also wouldn't know about any birthmarks. So, what do your legs look like?
Talia: Well, relative to the rest of my body, I guess they are long. . . . My thighs are wider than my hips—thanks, Mom—and you can see some dimples in them from cellulite, but that is mostly at the sides. And the back I bet if I turn around. Yup, there it is . . .

This step-by-step approach commonly has patients start with their heads and then move body part by body part (as instructed by the therapist) down to their toes. This approach to mirror exposure is commonly referred to as guided mirror exposure (Griffen, Naumann, & Hildebrandt, 2018). It also is sometimes called nonjudgmental mirror exposure and may be combined with mindfulness training.

Pure Versus Guided Mirror Exposure: Considerations

Limited research compares pure versus guided mirror exposure, and, as for mirror exposure generally, most studies include few if any male participants (Griffen et al., 2018). Nonetheless, results of the existing research suggest that both approaches to mirror exposure increase positive thoughts and reduce negative thoughts about the body. Pure mirror exposure, however, may confer additional benefit in reducing body dissatisfaction and possibly distress about body image (Griffen et al., 2018; Moreno-Dominguez et al., 2012). Pure mirror exposure, although initially conceptualized as following the habituation model, also may fit better with the inhibitory learning approach in that there is an explicit focus on tolerating distressing emotions about the body.

It is important to note that, to our knowledge, no research has directly tested at-home mirror exposure versus in-session exposure for either approach. The inhibitory learning perspective, however, suggests that conducting mirror exposure in as many different settings as possible would be optimal. So if you start in session, make sure to assign home-based mirror exposure, as anticipated by Talia. Depending on your patient, you may need one or more in-session exposures before moving to home practice. Assigning home practice only works if your patients are willing to actually do mirror exposure on their own, but our experience is that they are usually ready to try that after the first session. Under the inhibitory learning approach, it is actually a misnomer to refer to it as "home practice," as you want your patient to undertake practice in as many places as possible (e.g., at friends' homes; in front of different mirrors at home; walking down the street past many large shop windows; going between clothes stores and using the mirrors in changing rooms).

Mirror exposure, using either approach, also could be potentially enhanced by changing other features of the exposure. Examples of potential changes include wearing make-up versus not wearing make-up, wearing hair in more and less preferred ways, minimal clothing versus tight clothing versus no clothing (the latter should only be done in appropriate settings), deliberately including clothing that is less flattering, wearing gender-conforming versus gender nonconforming clothing. You can also vary the context in other ways, such as having patients conduct mirror exposure after eating anxiety-provoking foods or using interoceptive exercises to induce feared body sensations of fullness/bloating (see Chapter 15). Note that none of these have been tested experimentally, but all are consistent with how anxiety therapists approach exposure from an inhibitory learning framework.

Cognitive Dissonance-Based Mirror Exposure

A third method for conducting mirror exposure is the cognitive dissonance-based approach to mirror exposure. Cognitive dissonance is an uncomfortable psychological state that occurs when actions and beliefs are misaligned (Festinger, 1962). The dissonance approach to changing body image presumes that individuals have internalized culturally based appearance standards, which then increase body dissatisfaction. Theoretically, dissonance-based mirror exposure involves rejecting those standards by appreciating one's body while looking in a mirror as opposed to using the mirror as a tool for correction or critique in pursuit of the appearance ideal. Presumably, using the mirror in this new positive way (in a self-affirmation manner vs. with the goal of striving for the appearance ideal) decreases investment in appearance ideals, which then shifts body dissatisfaction. Changing how one uses mirrors may also alter mirror-based body-checking behaviors for some individuals.

Originally developed as a component of a highly researched ED prevention/body image improvement program (i.e., the Body Project; see Becker & Stice, 2017, for review), the dissonance approach instructs participants to say and write down 10 to 15 positive things, including at least several appearance features, while looking in a full-length mirror wearing little to no clothing. You can give your patients examples if you use this approach. For instance, make it clear that your patient can note things that she likes about her personality (e.g., her sense of humor), the functionality of her body (e.g., the way her legs let her run), and her appearance (e.g., the shape of her hips). She must include at least several appearance items, however, since these are likely to promote greater dissonance. This approach has not been tested as a stand-alone technique in a published study but is a component of a dissonance-based, or counterattitudinal, treatment for EDs (Stice, Rohde, Butryn, Menke, & Marti, 2015). Additionally, there is evidence from an analogue study that cognitive dissonance-based mirror exposure may yield more satisfaction with body image as compared to nonjudgmental/guided mirror exposure (Luethcke, McDaniel, & Becker, 2011).

Dissonance-based mirror exposure is typically assigned as homework right from the start. Although anecdotal evidence indicates that people do find dissonance-based mirror exposure quite challenging, it is likely less challenging than guided or pure mirror exposure, which makes it more suitable for home use quickly. Dissonance mirror exposure also may serve as a stepping stone to other forms of mirror exposure in patients who are otherwise unwilling to engage in mirror exposure.

Combining Multiple Mirror Exposure Approaches

A final way to conduct mirror exposure, one that is highly consistent with the inhibitory learning approach, albeit largely untested, would be to alternate between multiple approaches to conducting mirror exposure (see Lewer, Kosfelder, Michalak, Schroeder, Nasrawi, & Vocks, 2017, for an example of this strategy as part of a larger body image intervention). It is important to note that we do not currently know exactly how mirror exposure works (Griffen et al., 2018). As previously noted, both guided and pure mirror exposure appear to work even though they differ substantially in how they are conducted. Further, evidence from nonclinical research suggests that both positive (i.e., focusing on liked features) and negative (i.e., focusing on disliked body parts) mirror exposure produce improvements in body image (Jansen, Voorwinde, et al., 2016).

The success of different approaches to mirror exposure suggests that there likely are multiple pathways by which mirror exposure can act (see Griffen et al., 2018, for additional discussion). As noted in earlier chapters, exposure works when your patients learn what they need to learn, but different patients have different learning needs. It is entirely possible that the different approaches to mirror exposure are better and worse at teaching patients different things. Alternating between styles of mirror exposure would not only provide different ways to learn different things from mirror exposure; it also would be consistent with the inhibitory learning model's focus on increasing variability and decreasing predictability over time. For instance, after getting used to mirror exposure, your patient could agree to not knowing which type of mirror exposure will be used during a given exposure session. This could happen even in home-based mirror exposure with some planning (e.g., give your patient several envelopes, each containing a note indicating a different approach to exposure).

It is also important to note that no research currently suggests that the different approaches are mutually exclusive. It may, in fact, be beneficial for many patients to learn to look at their whole body and experience and tolerate the full range of thoughts and feelings that emerge, *and* to learn to objectively describe their body in a systematic manner, *and* to learn to identify things that they like about their body while looking at the mirror, thereby rejecting the common tendency to engage solely in self-disparaging dialogue in front of mirrors. In summary, although mirror exposure does have empirical support, many questions remain as to the optimal way to conduct mirror exposure. However, given that pure mirror exposure appears slightly more efficacious than the other forms (Griffen et al., 2018) and is also the most parsimonious approach of the three, we suggest you make pure mirror exposure your default approach and use your discretion as to when to introduce the others, if at all. As with all forms of exposure therapy, you will want to carefully assess your patients' short- and long-term response to mirror exposure in determining their needs.

Important Additional Considerations in Mirror Exposure

There are several additional factors to consider with mirror exposure. First is the use of this technique in patients who typically overuse mirrors to engage in body checking (which is a safety behavior designed to reduce anxiety). Mirror exposure has been found to reduce body checking in various studies (Griffen et al., 2018; Jansen, Voorwinde, et al., 2016). Nonetheless, Fairburn (2008) recommends limiting use of mirrors in patients who overuse them in daily life. It is important to realize that this recommendation is not incompatible with the use of exposure as previously outlined. When patients overuse mirrors on a regular basis to scrutinize their bodies, they are using the mirror in a manner that reduces short-term anxiety, thereby limiting improved distress tolerance. In the long term, this increases body dissatisfaction. In contrast, mirror exposure (using one or more of the previously described strategies) is designed to teach patients to use mirrors in a different way and to increase tolerance of distress around the body. As such, you may find it initially helpful to limit the use of mirrors only to tasks that necessitate their use (e.g., shaving one's face or putting on make-up) per Fairburn's (2008) recommendation *and* still implement mirror exposure. Note that this is akin to telling your patients to stop weighing themselves outside of therapy while still using open weighing in session for weight exposure.

In addition, you should consider who will conduct exposure (if it is conducted in session) and how much or what type of clothing your patient will wear. Mirror exposure often is conducted with patients wearing very revealing clothing, such as a swimsuit or even undergarments. You need to take care to avoid any sense of impropriety and consider the impact of both gender identity and sexual orientation in deciding who will conduct in-session mirror exposure. As an example, when working with female patients, it is appropriate for male therapists to ask patients to engage in mirror exposure while dressed in clothes they would wear normally or for physical activity in a public place. For patients with a history of sexual assault, you will need to take extra care in making sure they both fully consent to and feel in control of the decision to participate in mirror exposure. They also need to feel in control of the process of mirror exposure and the clothes they wear.

Some writers have voiced concerns about the use of mirror exposure with patients who are in higher weight bodies or who are at very low weights secondary to inadequate intake (e.g., Griffen et al., 2018). As previously noted, if you have patients who need to gain weight, it makes clinical sense to proceed with exposure after the majority of weight gain has occurred. These patients need to learn to tolerate their bodies at the weight where their bodies settle when they are engaging in appropriate eating. There is a dearth of research exploring the use of mirror exposure in low-weight patients. Thus, it is unclear if mirror exposure helps low-weight patients gain weight or whether exposure will produce the undesired effect of encouraging underweight patients to stay at a low weight instead of gaining needed weight. But what about higher weight patients? Should you use mirror exposure with them?

While the research is limited, it is clear that mirror exposure is effective for noneating-disordered obese individuals (Jansen et al., 2008). However, clinicians are often reluctant to use this approach when their patient is of higher weight. One suggested rationale for limiting mirror exposure with higher weight patients is that increased body satisfaction might demotivate patients from engaging in medically useful weight-loss efforts (Griffen et al., 2018). This, however, is a shaky rationale. Despite the widespread belief among both laypersons and healthcare providers that body dissatisfaction is associated with successful efforts to lose weight, research suggests that disliking one's body is associated with weight *gain* and use of unhealthy weight control behaviors over time (e.g., Neumark-Sztainer, Paxton, Hannan, Haines, & Story, 2006; Van den Berg, Neumark-Sztainer, Hannan, & Haines, 2007). By definition, ED patients have demonstrated a propensity to adopt extremely unhealthy eating (and, in many cases weight, management) behaviors. As such, as long as the patient is not underweight (see previous discussion), we argue that helping patients accept their weight wherever it falls when they are eating appropriately is the best course of action. Mirror exposure should not be withheld from patients whose biological make-up predisposes them to a socially undesirable weight. We, as clinicians, do not want to contribute to weight stigma.

It also is important to note that, to our knowledge, no research currently exists on mirror exposure with non-cisgender patients with EDs. The experience of the body may be substantially more complicated for transgender and nonbinary individuals. Thus, in the absence of any research that provides guidelines as to how to conduct mirror exposure in these populations, we suggest that particular care should be taken in how mirror exposure is used. We do not recommend removing this effective strategy entirely from your toolkit, but you will want to carefully think through (and openly discuss with your patient) the goals of mirror exposure and the approach used. You and your patient also need to collaboratively consider whether there are any potential drawbacks or possible unintended consequences for your patient related to their perception of their body as it relates to their gender identity.

Lastly, it is important to remember that the appearance ideal in many countries is a White appearance ideal. Thus, body image concerns among racial and ethnic minority patients may be more complex compared to White patients. For instance, during pure mirror exposure, Talia, who was White, initially focused excessively on her hair to avoid looking at the rest of her body. Talia's therapist appropriately encouraged Talia to look at her whole body and to focus on parts of her body that did not conform to the appearance ideal to increase her anxiety and distress. Jamilla, a Black patient in treatment for BN, similarly initially focused on her curly short hair. However, Jamilla wanted long, straight, "silky" hair and lighter skin in addition to a slimmer body, so as to better conform to the appearance ideal. For Jamilla, focusing on her hair created significant distress. Had the therapist refocused Jamilla to solely focus on weight, she would have invalidated the degree to which racial issues played a role in Jamilla's experience of her body. Once again, there is a lack of research to guide clinical practice in this area. However, you should strive to create a clinical environment that will allow patients to fully experience all liked and disliked parts of their body and recognize that there are multiple ways in which society can stigmatize the body.

In Vivo and Imaginal Body Image Exposure

Like many people without EDs, patients with EDs commonly avoid a range of situations secondary to negative body image. Avoidance behaviors vary widely, but common ones include avoiding some, or even all, of the following: wearing form-fitting clothing, wearing clothing that will leave parts of the body exposed (e.g., swimsuits, short sleeves, shorts), exercising in public, eating (particularly high-energy foods) in public, going without make-up, wearing certain hair styles, sexual intimacy, social events, buying new clothes, hugging others, going out without wearing body-shaping undergarments, etc. These avoidance behaviors prevent patients from learning that they can tolerate their body-related distress, reduce it, and live more fulfilled and less constricted lives. Patients also may fail to learn important information about the size and nature of their bodies. As a result, it is critical to address avoidance behaviors using exposure. One particularly good strategy is in vivo exposure.

You will want to fully assess all the ways in which body image concerns constrain your patients' lives so you can design appropriate exposure tasks. In assessing the manner in which patients avoid due to body image anxiety, we suggest using a self-report questionnaire such as the Body Image Avoidance Questionnaire (Rosen, Srebnik, Saltzberg, and Wendt, 1991). Beyond self-report questionnaires, we have had good luck with asking our patients variations of the following question: "Because of your body image concerns, what do you feel you cannot do?" Note that some of the exposure tasks you may develop with your patients may include deliberately designing activities that will elicit negative comments from others.

> **Clinician:** So last week your body image exposure assignment was to just sit in your chair at work without perching. You were afraid someone at work would comment on your weight if you did this and that you wouldn't be able to tolerate your anxiety or any comments. So how did this go?
>
> **Talia:** I was really nervous about it all weekend. And per our agreement, I still wore my shaper, but I did just sit this week at work without perching. A few times, I did it automatically when people came in to my cubicle, but then I forced myself to just sit like I would at home.
>
> **Clinician:** So what did you learn? And how do you feel about doing this regularly?
>
> **Talia:** Well, I learned that I can tolerate my anxiety. And that it also went down over time, which I didn't think would happen. I actually stopped thinking about it at times and just focused on my work. I also learned that people at work are either too busy to notice or too nice to comment. Or both. So I am okay doing this from now on at work. But I am sure it would be different on the train where they have that bench seating. I am sure there is some jerk out there that would say something.
>
> **Clinician:** And so what if they did?
>
> **Talia:** I would be mortified. If they said it in a loud voice and everyone starts looking at me and thinking "that out-of-control fatty is taking up more space than she deserves . . ."
>
> **Clinician:** And how long is your train ride?
>
> **Talia:** Fifty-five minutes if the train is on time.
>
> **Clinician:** How does it make you feel to try and be as small as you can for the whole 55 minutes each way every day you go to work?
>
> **Talia:** Tired and I can't use the time the way other people do.
>
> **Clinician:** Does that seem fair or as though it is improving your quality of life? What would your body-positivity social media group say?
>
> **Talia:** That I deserve to take up space and sit on the train like everyone else.
>
> **Clinician:** So what do you think your next exposure assignment should be?

Talia: Damn. I knew you were going to do this. So I should sit normally on the train? Every time?
Clinician: Sounds like a great plan to me.
Talia: Ughhh. Okay, I will do it. But I am going to think about how I want to respond if someone does say something.
Clinician: That is fine, but just to be clear—what is your fear prediction for this exposure? What do you fear you are going to do?
Talia: I fear I am going to burst into tears and make a scene and then everyone is going to look at me with disgust. And when I see their faces, I am going to lose control and make an even bigger scene—a giant scene. I can't even stand to think about it . . .

Given our weight-stigmatizing culture and the freedom that many people feel in disparaging people who are fat, it is not surprising that Talia eventually did receive some rude comments. However, she discovered that she could tolerate her anxiety and was capable of not bursting into tears, losing control, and making a giant scene. She also gradually developed, with the help of her body-positivity group and therapist, a repertoire of responses to rude comments. She then practiced saying these assertively, first to her therapist and then on the periodic occasions when someone was rude.

Body image exposure is a very powerful tool, and you want to encourage your patients to live a full life that is not overly constrained by body image concerns. It is, however, important to remember that many patients will face some very inappropriate and, at times, outright hostile feedback (especially if very low or high weight). Patients may need some support in learning to respond to these social interactions in an appropriately assertive manner. One stepping stone, which Talia's therapist used, is for you to say the predicted mean things in a harsh tone. If you are in a practice with other therapists, you can also recruit a stand-in exposure therapist or to practice role plays for assertiveness training. Additionally, your patients may find it helpful to engage with the body-positive community, particularly the groups that do truly represent all sizes, shapes, races, ethnicities, genders, etc. These groups can also help patients navigate tricky social interactions and find support.

Talia ultimately completed exposure to returning to the gym, first wearing baggy clothes and then more form-fitting clothing. The latter could only happen after she completed exposure to trying on and buying the form-fitting clothing. She also completed exposure eating high-energy foods in front of friends, work colleagues, and a potential dating partner. She also went swimming wearing a bathing suit for the first time in a decade. Finally, Talia completed exposure to going to work without wearing body shaping undergarments and eventually discontinued use of these. Talia had particularly intense anxiety about forgoing her body-shaping undergarments and initially was unwilling to try this exposure assignment. As a result, she and her therapist first completed one session of *imaginal exposure* to Talia's most feared prediction of what would happen at work (see Chapter 15 for additional discussion of imaginal exposure).

> **Therapist:** Please close your eyes and imagine that you are showing up for work without your shaper. I want you to picture this as vividly as possible and then walk me through your most feared expectation.
> **Talia:** So I am walking into the office and the new woman who sits at the reception desk is totally shocked when she sees me. Her eyes get really big and her jaw drops open. Then she just starts laughing, and she picks up the phone. I don't know who she is calling but I know she is now laughing at me with someone.
> **Therapist:** Then what happens?
> **Talia:** I go to my desk and a little while later my co-worker Steve comes over. He's a total jerk. And he just looks down at me and smirks and says, "I had to see it for myself," and then walks away. I am so humiliated.
> **Therapist:** How much distress do you feel right now?
> **Talia:** Eighty-five.
> **Therapist:** And what happens next?
> **Talia:** I get a call. It is my boss. She wants to see me immediately. I go in to see her and she says that this is very awkward, but she has received complaints that I am not appropriately dressed today. She wants me to go home and dress the way I usually do. She also wants me to meet with HR to talk about the wellness program so I can start eating properly again and lose weight. So I leave and everyone is giggling. I know they know that my boss just sent me home.
> **Therapist:** Really well done. Please take me though it again . . .

After this imaginal work and a week of home practice using an audio recording of her in-session imaginal exposure, Talia was willing to begin in vivo exposure.

SUMMARY

Body image disturbances, which are characterized by elevated anxiety and avoidance, play a central role in the development and maintenance of EDs. Fortunately, exposure-based strategies, during which patients are encouraged to confront stimuli that evoke body-related anxiety, appear effective in reducing the cognitive, affective, and behavioral features of body image disturbances in EDs. In particular, mirror exposure is a body-focused treatment intervention that has amassed consistent empirical support in reducing various facets of body image distress. When implementing mirror exposure with your patients, there are several important things that you will need to consider. These include the type of mirror exposure you choose to use, the way you will encourage your patient to dress, and how you will address your patient's tendency to use mirrors to inappropriately scrutinize (i.e., check) her physique. To date, research has yet to provide definitive answers to these questions. So, for the time being, you will need to rely on your functional assessment and collaboratively make decisions with your patients. Aside from mirrors, your patients also are likely to describe a host of other anxiety-provoking stimuli (e.g., wearing "revealing" clothing items) that will be important for you to incorporate into your patients' exposure work.

14

Emotion-Focused and Interpersonal Exposure

So far, we have considered exposure in EDs as it applies to the most central elements of eating pathology—food, eating, weight, and body image. However, EDs frequently also have interpersonal and emotional elements, and you often can use exposure to address these important maintaining factors as well. Indeed, interpersonal and emotional factors are frequently key drivers of residual bingeing and purging behaviors that have not responded to stabilization of eating behaviors. Given the importance of stopping such behaviors completely to reduce the risk of relapse (e.g., Keel, Dorer, Franko, Jackson, & Herzog (2005), you need to attend to those remaining binge–purge episodes. Further, in some cases (particularly some BED and ARFID cases, where starvation is not a key issue), emotional triggers may serve as the biggest driver of bingeing or food avoidance (e.g., anxiety in some cases of BED; disgust in some cases of ARFID). Remember, however, that emotional triggers are present across all ED diagnoses (e.g., McManus, Waller, & Chadwick, 1996). For instance, interpersonal and social triggers have been shown to drive bulimic behaviors in BN (e.g., Steiger, Gauvin, Jabalpurwala, Seguin, & Stotland, 1999). In addition, emotion and interpersonal factors may interact with other elements of EDs, including food cues and body image concerns.

Having said this, it also is important to remember that negative mood is usually not the first thing you will want to address when working with your ED patients, given that mood is often a *consequence* of ED behaviors rather than being a causal factor. For instance, many, if not most, of your patients will experience negative emotions secondary to engaging in bingeing and purging behaviors. Indeed, many patients report these behaviors are highly distressing, particularly after the event. In addition, the effects of starvation on serotonin levels (particularly carbohydrate deprivation, which can result in unstable mood) and the loss of positive reinforcers in life (e.g., friends, social interaction, development opportunities) can drive negative mood. Therefore, exposure to emotional and interpersonal states should follow, not precede, normalization of eating. This chapter is deliberately placed later in this section of the book, to reflect that prioritization.

> Tammy is 32-year-old woman who has experienced BN for most of the past 13 years, with only occasional periods of remission (e.g., during her two pregnancies and for a short time after each). In the first part of treatment, she has benefited from exposure for both eating and weight concerns. Tammy has stopped starving herself and no longer engages in any starvation-based bingeing with compensatory vomiting; previously she did this four times per week. However, Tammy still binges and vomits approximately once every 2 weeks, despite having no hunger or craving experiences that would explain these behaviors. The vomiting does not always follow the binge-eating. Tammy cannot make sense of why she binges and vomits, as she is unaware of any setting conditions or contingencies that might explain her behaviors.

In Tammy's case, behavioral chain analysis (Linehan, 1993) helped Tammy and her clinician to determine that the behaviors were driven by mood and interpersonal interactions, rather than the distress and social isolation being driven by having binged and purged.

> For binge eating, diaries of her eating and the underlying cognitions and emotions showed that Tammy binged without vomiting when she was anxious about the state of her relationship, and that the binge eating was followed by an immediate, short-term reduction in those emotions. However, in the longer term, the emotions returned, because binge eating did not address the situations that originally made her anxious. Further, they worsened her mood because she felt more isolated after having stayed alone to binge. In contrast, Tammy found that she was more likely to binge eat and vomit when she felt socially anxious and feared embarrassment in front of others. Again, the behavior reduced her social anxiety in the short term but resulted in greater embarrassment in the longer term.

Once the critical link is established (which usually requires that starvation effects are minimized in the earlier part of therapy), it is appropriate to use exposure to address some emotional states and interpersonal issues.

EXPOSURE TO EMOTIONS

Before you embark on exposure to emotions, you will first need to demonstrate to your patients the role that their emotions play in driving their ED behaviors. Then, it becomes possible to use exposure to address that association.

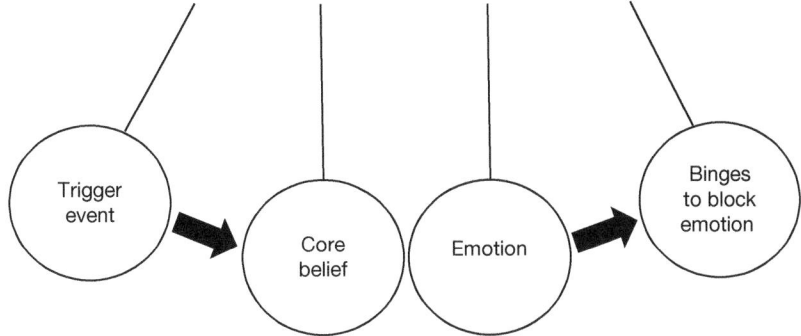

Figure 14.1. An illustration of the Newton's cradle model, as shared with Tammy.

Formulating the Role of Emotions for Your Patient

The Newton's cradle model (Waller et al., 2007; Waller, Turner, Tatham, Mountford, & Wade, 2019) can be used to formulate the role of emotions in the use of ED behaviors. In short, this model is a means of explaining to your patients that their behaviors have understandable causes. Very often, patients find it hard to identify why they restrict or use bulimic behaviors. Sometimes, they do not see any trigger or other factors that might explain why they engage in a behavior, which is when you will hear a patient like Tammy saying something like: "I suppose it is just a habit—I just do it."

Your first task is to use microanalysis of the specific behavior to demonstrate that there are, in fact, specific reasons that your patient does something. This is where you can introduce the Newton's cradle analogy, which will help you hypothesize with Tammy that there are understandable reasons for her behavior. Figure 14.1 illustrates the Newton's cradle, where the trigger (e.g., a life event) activates core beliefs, which, in turn, activate an emotional state. Where Tammy is avoidant of emotions or wishes to "block" them once they are activated, then a behavior such as bingeing can result, all very rapidly and without immediate conscious processing:

You will see that the core task is to link triggers, cognitions (usually core beliefs), emotions, and behavior, showing Tammy that these can all happen in a very short period of time and can be brought to awareness when she knows what she is looking for.

> **Clinician:** So, we know that you are still bingeing occasionally and that it is not because you are starved. What do you think causes the binges now?
> **Tammy:** Well, I have been doing it so long now that I think it is just habit. Maybe I have a few minutes, and I just eat to fill the time?
> **Clinician:** I can see that might seem like the obvious label to put on it, but I want us to look at what was going on and see if we can explain your binges in a way that makes sense and lets you learn how to challenge

and stop them. I think that there might be a sort of chain of events that happens each time, but it all happens so fast that you have no time to process it. Do you know what a Newton's cradle is?

Tammy: You mean that set of balls hanging from strings, where you let the first one go and the last one pops up, but the ones in the middle stay still?

Clinician: That's the one. I want to see if we can explain your behavior of bingeing as being the last ball in that chain, where all the rest comes so fast that you need help to be able to see it, so that you can learn to stop it. Let's draw it out. . . . Imagine a Newton's Cradle with four of those balls. The first ball in the chain is the trigger—what started it all. Then the next one is the beliefs that the trigger activates. The third ball is the emotion that your beliefs trigger. Then you get to the final ball—your bingeing, which you use to avoid or reduce that emotional state. Does that make sense?

Tammy: I suppose it could, but what would be going on for me?

Clinician: Well, we would need to get you to keep a diary to be sure, but let's hypothesize, so that we know what you might look at when you get the urge to binge. You have talked about an emotion that happens around the time that you binge—feeling anxious—though you did not see any connection at the time. Maybe what is going on is that something makes you feel anxious, and you have learned that if you binge, then that emotion goes away for a bit.

Tammy: That would be the third and fourth balls then?

Clinician: You got it. So what situations make you more likely to be anxious when that happens—that first ball? What was happening the last time that you binged?

Tammy: On Friday? I binged around 9 PM. I had spent ages waiting for my boyfriend to turn up to take me out. We had arranged it. He finally messaged me at about 8.30 PM to tell me that he had gone out with his mates instead—he does that a lot.

Clinician: So if that happened to a friend, what would you think she might be feeling when she got the message?

Tammy: Well, it has happened a few times to my pal Julie, and she always gets really worried that her boyfriend is losing interest in her. She usually dumps the man very soon after that, for letting her down.

Clinician: Do you think that you might have been feeling the same thing—anxious? But that you might not be used to thinking about that sort of feeling or even block it out by using bingeing?

Tammy: I suppose it is possible. I do sort of fear that my boyfriend might get sick of me and leave me. I get nervous talking to new people, so I fear having to find someone new to date. But why do I binge, where Julie can just blame the man and dump him?

Clinician: That is where the second ball comes in—that core belief. We all have beliefs about what sort of person we are, what we deserve, and so on. I wonder if you grew up in a home that meant that showing and feeling emotions is not acceptable or safe? How did your family react if you got upset when you were young?

Tammy: Ooh. We *never* showed anything like that. Mum and Dad were always very definite—the rule was to keep everything happy and not to make a fuss, whatever was going on. I could never tell them something that was outside of that, like when I was bullied at school. Even now, I could never tell them that my boyfriend cheated on me a couple of times.

Clinician: It sounds like the pattern of thinking in the second ball includes two beliefs. The first would be a belief that your boyfriend is getting sick of you, which makes you anxious. The second, termed an "emotional inhibition" core belief is that you are not allowed to experience or show negative emotions, and it is common when you grow up in what is called an "emotionally invalidating" environment like the one that you are describing there.

Tammy: That is a thing? I thought it was just how things are.

Clinician: Everyone has core beliefs and emotions—yours just seem to be interacting with the world as it is now to result in you using binges. So, it sounds like the trigger on Friday was your boyfriend treating you in a way that activated your emotional inhibition beliefs. Even though you were anxious, you could not express or even experience the emotion, and you binged as a way of stopping that emotional experience. But you need to see if that is right for you and whether it works in other situations. So it is time to get you to do a diary whenever you get the urge to binge, where you find out if there are links between those experiences, your core beliefs, your emotions, and your binges.

Tammy: That makes sense—my own Newton's cradle.

You will note that even talking about these links and the emotional element has the potential to be emotionally challenging for Tammy, so structuring matters this way may act as exposure, depending on the patient. If your patient is reluctant to consider her emotional experiences, then it is potentially beneficial to keep talking about those emotions (rather than backing off, for fear of distressing your patient) to extend the exposure to emotional states. Otherwise, you may inadvertently reinforce the safety/avoidant behavior of emotional avoidance.

Addressing Emotions Using Exposure

Obviously, there are many methods that can be used to address the behavioral chain captured by the Newton's cradle model. They can include changing the trigger (e.g., encourage Tammy to change the "rule" whereby her boyfriend can do as he wishes without consequences), addressing the core beliefs directly using cognitive techniques (e.g., cognitive restructuring), and behaviorally challenging the belief and associated emotions (e.g., encouraging Tammy to tell her boyfriend that he should just go out, to learn whether he really does lose interest in her). However, you will often find that exposure is also a useful tool to consider.

When deciding what strategy to use to address the behavioral chain, remember that exposure is largely considered a potent strategy for addressing anxiety and, to a somewhat lesser degree, disgust. It is not typically considered the best strategy for addressing some other negatively valenced emotions such as anger, sadness, and shame. However, it also is important to remember that many patients, like Tammy, are anxious about experiencing a wide range of negative emotions, and exposure is an excellent strategy for addressing that anxiety about experiencing emotions. For instance, suppose that Tammy's boyfriend's behavior first and foremost made her extremely angry instead of anxious and that she used binge eating to manage her anger so that she does not physically attack him when he eventually comes home. Exposure is not a terribly good technique for reducing anger as it can promote anger rehearsal, which will increase the anger and make Tammy even more likely to attack (Linehan, 1993). Cognitive restructuring, assertiveness training, distraction, and/or comprehensive anger management training (in the case of profound, functionally impairing anger) all would likely be better strategies for altering problematic anger. Yet, if Tammy finds it very anxiety provoking to get appropriately angry at her boyfriend's insensitive behavior (possibly because she fears that it will lead her to behave in a way that will make her boyfriend leave or because her childhood made her fear negative emotions generally), and she uses binge eating, restriction, or vomiting to manage her anxiety about getting angry, then you will want to consider using exposure to address that anxiety about experiencing negative emotions.

To use exposure to address ED behaviors triggered by your patients' emotional experiences, you will need to work with them to identify the activation and nature of the emotion (or emotional cascade in the case that a negative emotion such as anger triggers anxiety). You also will need to identify the way in which ED behaviors are functionally related to the emotion. Finally, you will need to consider if the emotion is one that likely can be successfully addressed with exposure.

Rather than giving our patients a long list of emotion terms to figure out what they are feeling, we find that we are usually able to hypothesize what the key emotions are based on the situation (e.g., Tammy's response to her uncaring boyfriend was mostly likely to be anxious, angry, or sad about being rejected). We openly share these hypotheses with our patients to see which ones (if any) seem to fit for them. We also discuss common signs of the hypothesized emotion(s). For instance, Tammy described feeling flushed and "jittery" whenever she had this experience with her boyfriend. Therefore, whenever she had the urge to binge eat, Tammy was asked to identify whether that trigger and those physical signs were present.

Having identified the key functional relationships between the trigger, emotion, and ED behavior, the next step for you is to discuss with your patient how she might undertake the necessary exposure work. To do this, you will need to identify safety behaviors your patient uses to manage her emotions (e.g., Tammy usually made sure she had several movies recorded to watch so she could say she had something else just as good to do if her boyfriend canceled, and she also used binge eating to reduce her anxiety). You also will need to determine if your patient is using avoidance (e.g., Tammy tried to guess which nights her boyfriend would want to spend with his friends, and she never asked to go out on those nights).

Initially, Tammy's clinician worked with the anxiety-triggered binge behavior by giving Tammy the task of sitting with her anxiety for at least 45 minutes before actively deciding whether she wanted to binge. Tammy struggled to identify her harm expectancy about feeling anxious ("I was just taught you should not feel negative emotions") so her clinician set up the exposure as a chance to learn that she could tolerate feeling anxious without engaging in binge eating. If Tammy had been reluctant to engage in pure exposure of this form at the outset (or if it seemed unlikely that Tammy would be able to resist binge eating), the clinician could have instructed her to use distraction methods to help her resist the urge to binge (e.g., Tammy might be encouraged to talk to a friend about other issues or to paint her nails). This, however, should be seen only as a step toward pure exposure, as such distraction will dampen the effect of the exposure. Similarly, anxiety reduction methods such as relaxation, mindfulness meditation, etc. should be avoided as far as possible, as they are likely to dampen the effect of exposure even more.

Once Tammy's clinician realized that Tammy was retreating from asking anything of her boyfriend on certain nights so as to avoid triggering her anxiety, and she was still falling back on binge eating to address other emotions (e.g., loneliness, disappointment, envy of her friends who had something to do on Friday night), she proposed to Tammy that she engage in exposure to possibly being rejected by her boyfriend. For instance, the clinician encouraged Tammy to ask him to take her out on a "friends night" and resist any change in plans. This gave Tammy the chance to test out her fear prediction that (a) her boyfriend would break up with her and (b) that she would be unable to tolerate the breakup or, even, his being annoyed with her for requiring him to treat her with respect. By triggering the trigger in this way, you give Tammy the chance to learn the link between her boyfriend's behavior and her emotion and to experience exposure on a timescale that is more controllable (rather than potentially having to wait weeks for the chance to learn). This is an example of exposing the patient to an interpersonal situation, which we discuss further in the next section.

EXPOSURE TO INTERPERSONAL EVALUATION

A variety of interpersonal situations also are capable of triggering bulimic or restrictive behavior through their impact on cognitive and emotional experiences (via the previously discussed Newton's cradle model). While such issues have already been addressed to some degree in Tammy's case (e.g., the uncaring boyfriend), it is important to note one particularly common emotional response that can be a trigger to pathological eating behaviors, and which Tammy is also reporting—social anxiety. It is worth noting that elevated social anxiety has been found to diminish the benefit that patients receive from treatment for their ED (Smith et al., 2018).

Tammy reports that she is binge eating and vomiting when she feels socially anxious and fearful of being embarrassed. You will often find it relatively easy to identify such triggers, as your patient is likely to be able to identify both that she feels anxious and the fear of negative evaluation that underpins that emotion. However, such identification can be made harder in some cases. Patients like Tammy can develop a long-standing pattern of socially avoidant behaviors that can mean that the beliefs and emotions are not apparent to her or to you. Thus, throughout treatment, you should assess your patient's life, considering whether social anxiety is a possible explanation of a limited social life and friendship circle (e.g., a patient who has stayed with their parents well into adulthood or who has few or no friends).

In a case such as Tammy's, you might consider exposure in the following ways with the aim of your patients learning (a) improved tolerance of anxiety and (b) that safety behaviors and avoidance are ineffective in the long term. In keeping with the inhibitory learning approach, this involves a range of experiences in different settings and aims for the highest tolerable level of anxiety:

- Entering a range of scary social situations (e.g., going out to new situations, where there is unpredictability);
- Engaging with strangers as well as known people (e.g., going somewhere such as a coffee shop and talking to strangers);
- Exposure to embarrassment (e.g., deliberately doing something foolish in front of other people to discover that embarrassment fades and is more tolerable than is often imagined);
- Reduction in avoidant behaviors (e.g., refraining from using alcohol to reduce anxiety at social gatherings); a
- Not using distractors (e.g., not checking her phone all the time)

Interpersonal Evaluation During Eating

Fear of social evaluation is common in eating scenarios. Patients may not only fear eating in front of other people and being scrutinized; they may also fear that other people will comment on what they eat. One method for addressing this is to engage in structured exposure with the therapist, both to scrutiny by another person and to negative comments. Exposure can later be expanded to other people, optimally as quickly as feasible. Vitousek (Becker, Waller & Vitousek, 2018) has probably honed this approach to the greatest degree. In the following discussion, we present a sample hierarchy of steps for engaging in this type of exposure with dessert food. However, you could start with different foods depending on what is relevant for a given patient and depending on what that patient is willing to undertake. You can also titrate steps according to patient willingness. Identifying the comments (and possibly nonverbal expressions) that your patient most fears will help you tailor the exposure so that she is ultimately exposed to her most feared combination of comments and food. As per the inhibitory learning model, over time this approach should be practiced with other people, in different settings, and with different foods.

> **A Method for Mixed Interpersonal and Food Exposure: Hierarchy of Steps**
>
> - Therapist and patient each order a dessert at a restaurant. Therapist orders big elaborate dessert, and patient orders small dish of ice cream with no toppings.
> - Therapist orders big dessert, and patient orders ice cream with toppings.
> - Therapist orders big dessert, and patient orders ice cream with toppings. Therapist comments on both desserts having a lot of calories and fat.
> - Therapist and patient both order big desserts, and therapist comments on calories. Therapist also wonders aloud about the possibility of patient gaining weight as a result of eating the dessert.
> - Therapist orders ice cream with toppings, and patient orders big elaborate dessert. Therapist comments on calories and potential for weight gain.
> - Therapist orders plain ice cream, and patient orders big elaborate dessert. Therapist makes negative comments about patient eating that big a dessert.

SUMMARY

This chapter has addressed the range of ways in which exposure can be used to address emotional and related interpersonal triggers to ED behaviors. The Newton's cradle model will allow you to formulate such events, using behavioral chain analysis to understand behaviors that we often hear described as "just a habit." Such an understanding means that you can break open the steps in that chain to intervene. While there are several potential points and methods that can be used for such an intervention, the use of exposure to address the emotional states directly will give you a powerful tool to get the maximum effect in a relatively short time by preventing avoidant and safety behaviors. Doing exposure work that combines interpersonal and eating concerns can be particularly potent.

15
Novel Ways to Use Exposure for Eating Disorders

The aim of this chapter is to consider three additional forms of exposure that can be useful in augmenting treatment for EDs—interoceptive approaches, imaginal exposure, and exposure for addressing magical thinking. Note that these forms of exposure should be considered relatively experimental in the treatment of EDs in that they lack significant empirical support as supplemental strategies for EDs. However, each is widely used in the treatment of anxiety-based disorders, and the parallels between the EDs and those disorders are quite evident. Moreover, the proposed use of these methods for treating EDs is not entirely novel. All have either been proposed by other authors (e.g., Boswell, Anderson, & Anderson, 2015; Levinson, Rapp, & Riley, 2014) and/or used clinically by the present authors. However, there is a lot more experimental evidence needed for all of the following.

INTEROCEPTIVE EXPOSURE

As noted in Chapter 2, interoceptive exposure is most commonly used with panic disorder. However, researchers are increasingly focusing on its potential as a transdiagnostic intervention. For instance, interoceptive exposure has been incorporated into the treatment of other anxiety-based disorders, such as social anxiety disorder, generalized anxiety disorder, and PTSD (Boswell et al., 2013; Wald & Taylor, 2007).

Potential Utility With Eating Disorders

Researchers are increasingly finding that interoceptive sensitivity to physical sensations is not limited to sensations associated with anxiety. Rather, it extends to physical sensations associated with a wide array of emotional and psychophysical responses, including hunger and satiety (Boswell et al., 2015; Herbert, Muth, Pollatos, & Herbert, 2012; Merwin, Zucker, Lacy, & Elliott, 2010). Indeed, patients with EDs regularly report problems with physical sensations (particularly those related to eating). Researchers have distinguished two specific concerns that present in EDs: (a) lack of clarity or confusion about physical sensations (i.e., interoceptive cues) and (b) intolerance or lack of acceptance of interoceptive cues (e.g., fullness) and their associated emotional states (e.g., anxiety, guilt, disgust; see Boswell et al., 2015, for additional conceptual discussion of interoceptive exposure and EDs).

The former problem (lack of clarity about physical sensations) is most obviously demonstrated by patients who (a) complain about having a full stomach after eating very little food and then (b) point to their lower abdomen when asked to show you where their stomach is, thus missing the location of their real stomach by up to 12 inches. In this case, our patients are undoubtedly experiencing physical sensations following eating, but they are likely demonstrating anxiety rather than fullness. Patients' reactions to these anxiety sensations (and the reaction of the clinicians who fail to check the details of their experience) is commonly to "stop eating in case my stomach bursts." However, an exposure therapy approach would be to "keep eating and learn that the sensations in your abdomen go away as you learn you can tolerate your anxiety." Over time, patients also can learn the actual sensations associated with their stomach itself actually being full.

The latter concern (intolerance of those physical sensations) most clearly maps onto the way in which interoceptive exposure is typically used in the treatment of panic and anxiety-based disorders and is the focus of the following two case examples.

> Lucia had a 3-year history of BN. Despite making significant progress with increasing the frequency of her meals, she continued to eat small amounts of food at each meal because she could not "stand to feel full." Lucia and her therapist designed three exposure tasks to increase Lucia's tolerance of feeling full as well as the anxiety that accompanied feeling full. First, they started with an in-session meal that consisted of Lucia's typical lunch—a small turkey sandwich and an apple. However, before eating the meal, Lucia quickly drank two large glasses of water. By the time she finished her meal, she reported very high levels of "fullness" and anxiety regarding this sensation. Lucia's therapist had her focus on the sensations of fullness, the sense that her clothing was tighter than normal, and her fear that the fullness indicated she would gain a significant amount of weight. Importantly, Lucia did not just fear gaining weight; she also reported being unable to tolerate the anxiety associated with her fear of weight gain. After repeating this exposure daily for a week, Lucia increased the interoceptive sensations by wearing shapewear that put considerable pressure on her abdomen to increase the tight clothing sensations. One week later, Lucia agreed to increasing the size of her lunch meal as her next exposure assignment. She noted that she had learned the sensation of fullness was more tolerable than she thought and that it also was less predictive of weight gain than expected.

> Tomás, who avoided a variety of foods he feared would cause choking, reported that whenever he tried to eat feared foods, his heart would start racing and it would feel like his throat was closing. Tomás reported hating these sensations and interpreted them as meaning that the food really was dangerous to consume. Tomás's therapist had him complete traditional panic disorder interoceptive exposure activities because these sensations are also commonly reported by patients with EDs. Tomás's therapist first had Tomás complete a testing round of several physical exercises, so as to discover which ones most reliably produced the heart-racing and throat-closing sensations that Tomás associated with eating feared foods. For instance, Tomás hyperventilated, ran in place, spun around in circle, breathed through a small straw, and tensed his body. Each testing exercise lasted for approximately 1 minute. Several exercises increased his heart rate, but Tomás reported the sensations associated with hyperventilation and straw-breathing were more anxiety provoking. He noted that because exercise-induced heart racing (i.e., running in place) was to be expected, he did not find it anxiety provoking. Tomás was then assigned hyperventilation and straw-breathing homework for a week. When he returned to his next session, Tomás reported neither exercise bothered him significantly. Subsequently, he became more willing to engage in exposure to feared foods.

Note that spinning in a chair and tensing the body are not commonly viewed as exercises that will increase heart-rate or throat-closing sensations. However, you will find that it can be hard to predict exactly which exercises will produce the right combination of feared sensations in the right manner for a specific individual. As it turned out, Tomás didn't fear heart racing (or shortness of breath) when it could be attributed to "exercise." For this reason, if you are going to use interoceptive exposure, consider testing a range of exercises. You may be surprised which ones your patient finds most aversive.

In addition to the traditional panic disorder interoceptive exercises, Boswell, Anderson, and Anderson (2015) proposed the following strategies for inducing physiological sensations that can be distressing for ED patients:

> - Drinking a large amount of water, which produces sensations of fullness;
> - Wearing tight clothing, which increases a sense of constriction;
> - Smelling or tasting foods that are associated with eating;
> - Bouncing up and down or moving in a way to make the body jiggle;
> - Sitting close to someone, which creates a sensation of being touched;
> - Sitting or lying on a beanbag or blow-up chair, so that the body feels heavy;
> - Wearing clothing that is damp, which increases the tactile nature of clothing;
> - Sitting on a hard, flat surface, so thighs and buttocks spread; and
> - Pushing out the belly, which makes it look and feel larger.

As demonstrated in both the cases of Lucia and Tomás, interoceptive exposure can be used to address sensations that create a barrier to proceeding with eating exposure. Interoceptive exposure can also be combined with other forms of exposure, including weighing and body image exposure. Further, as per the inhibitory learning model, if you combine these forms of exposure over time (i.e., layering), you are likely to strengthen safety learning. For this reason, after Tomás completed successful exposure to a new food, his therapist had him engage in hyperventilation or straw-breathing before eating the food. Tomás eventually adopted the exposure lifestyle and decided to hyperventilate, breathe through the straw, and then eat his feared food. Similarly, Lucia pushed herself to wear shapewear after introducing pizza back into her diet. She noted that eating pizza while wearing something very tight created substantially more anxiety than eating pizza when her clothing was loose, even though she knew the calorie content did not change.

IMAGINAL EXPOSURE

Imaginal exposure for EDs is one of the more newly proposed forms of exposure for EDs. However, as noted by Levinson et al. (2014), who first suggested the use of imaginal exposure to address fear of fatness in AN, imaginal exposure has a very long history of use in the treatment of anxiety-based disorders to address fearful situations that cannot be recreated or accessed in vivo. For instance, imaginal exposure has been used in the treatment of PTSD to expose patients to fear-provoking memories of traumatic events (Foa & Rothbaum, 1998). Imaginal exposure also has a long history in both OCD treatment, where it is used to complete exposure to obsessional images or future feared outcomes (Stanley & Averill, 1998), and GAD treatment, for worry exposure (Zinbarg, Craske, & Barlow, 1993). Similarly, imaginal exposure can be used to address future feared outcomes (e.g., gaining an extreme amount of weight, being abandoned for gaining weight) that serve as core maintaining fears in EDs.

Potential Utility With Eating Disorders

Although use of imaginal exposure for EDs is very new and only supported to date by a case study and an online open trial (Levinson et al., 2014, 2017), it is highly consistent with the ways in which anxiety therapists address fears that cannot be addressed in real life for anxiety-based disorders. Imaginal exposure can be conducted in a number of ways. First, if your patient has a clear image or predicted outcome, they may be able to simply tell you what is happening using the present tense and trying to imagine it very clearly. For instance, Tyra, who was being treated for OCD, had a very clear image of her younger brother being hit by a car. To reduce her anxiety, she constantly checked on him via texting, which impaired both of their attention in school. Because Tyra's image was very clear, she did not need to write it down.

> **Clinician:** So close your eyes and tell me what happens to your brother. Just walk me through it, trying to see it as clearly as you can in your head.
> **Tyra:** So Darrell is walking out of school, and it is a really busy pick-up time. He doesn't pay attention well because he is checking his phone. There is this area where the sidewalk blends with the street—no curb—so it is really easy to step into the street. Darrell just doesn't look—he never looks—and wanders into the street and I can see this big SUV just running right into him. The driver sees Darrell at the last minute but can't stop. He tries to swerve but it's too late. And I can see Darrell bouncing up off the front of the SUV, and there is blood and his body is at a funny angle, and he's not moving, and I just know my baby brother is dead.
> **Clinician:** And how much anxiety are you experiencing right now?
> **Tyra:** Ninety-five. I hate this.
> **Clinician:** I understand, but do you remember why we are doing this?
> **Tyra:** Because the images are not real and I can learn to tolerate them and then I won't be so bothered.
> **Clinician:** Please take me through it again . . .

Tyra subsequently listened to an audio recording of this session in multiple locations, all while inhibiting the urge to engage in the safety behavior to text her brother and confirm that he was alright. Like Tyra, patients with PTSD are often able to simply "walk" you through their traumatic memories. However, some patients need to write down the feared scenario to really identify the relevant details. In this case, your patient would read the scenario aloud.

This need to write out the situation may be true of many ED patients. The limited imaginal exposure research to date with EDs has involved patients writing out their feared scenario. For example, KC was reluctant to engage in eating regular meals in everyday life, so imaginal exposure was used to elicit the anxiety even though the food had not been eaten, to allow some safety learning to take place. Note that, per the inhibitory learning model, decreasing KC's fear to actually eating *before* starting actual eating exposure may make in vivo exposure somewhat less effective, compared to just getting KC to eat. This is because it may reduce the degree to which KC's harm expectancy is violated. However, KC's harm expectancy about becoming really fat and being abandoned by friends will never be violated if KC simply refuses to begin in vivo exposure.

> **Therapist:** So let's map out what you fear will happen if you eat regularly sized meals three times per day.
> **KC:** I think I am going to get really fat.
> **Therapist:** And what would be so bad about that?
> **KC:** Well, first I wouldn't be able to stand it (*shudders*). I would feel so gross seeing my stomach bulging and losing my slim arms and legs. I don't even want to think about having such fat arms and legs with the fat hanging everywhere.

Therapist: What else would be really bad?

KC: People who know me would judge me for the weight gain. They would think I was weak and lazy for letting this happen. I know some wouldn't want to be seen with me and would make up excuses for not seeing me.

Therapist: Okay, so let's write this down in as much detail as you can. Make it really vivid. Where are you, what do you see, what do you feel emotionally, who are you with? Include specific thoughts.

After KC developed their scenario, the therapist had them read it out loud repeatedly. Based on imaginal exposure for other disorders, KC and their therapist made an audio recording of KC reading the scenario over and over, so that KC could listen to it in many different settings.

EXPOSURE FOR "MAGICAL THINKING"

Magical thinking is a common experience in some anxiety disorders. For example, many OCD patients experience *thought–action fusion,* where they fear that thinking about a bad outcome is likely to make that outcome happen (e.g., imagining a relative being seriously ill is likely to make that illness happen), even though there is no realistic mechanism whereby that would happen. Similarly, superstitious thinking is present in many anxious patients (e.g., "Putting my socks on in the right order is vital, or bad things will happen to me").

Potential Utility With Eating Disorders

ED patients periodically engage in magical thinking. Magical thinking consists of beliefs that do not make logical sense but nonetheless lead to avoidant or safety behaviors to reduce anxiety. A key example is thought–shape fusion (Shafran & Robinson, 2004), in which patients believe that simply thinking about food can make them gain weight (akin to thought–action fusion in OCD), but there are many others, as detailed here:

> **Examples of Magical Thinking in EDs**
>
> - Belief that calories will transfer to the body if one merely looks at or smells high calorie foods, such as dessert
> - Belief that being close to a person of higher weight will lead one to gain weight, because weight will magically transfer from one person to another
> - Fear that there is a meaningful number of calories in toothpaste that will be consumed during teeth brushing

- Fear that calories will be absorbed through the skin from flavored lip moisturizers or scented body lotions
- Fear that a single food item (e.g., piece of pizza) will cause implausible weight gain (e.g., 10 pounds)
- Fear that missing a day of planned exercise will result in substantial changes to physique (e.g., noticeable loss of muscle tone)

Such beliefs are key to understanding why so many patients with EDs experience a profound fear of uncontrollable weight gain (Waller & Mountford, 2015).

One of the fastest approaches to treating magical thinking is to use exposure to violate the harm expectancy, teaching your patients that they can tolerate the anxiety that accompanies a decrease in avoidant and safety behaviors.

Shelby believed that touching high-calorie foods would result in her absorbing the calories through her skin. She was not only unwilling to eat high-calorie foods but refused to be in the same room as high-calorie foods out of fear that she would accidentally touch the food and absorb calories. Shelby's exposure started with sitting in her therapist's office with a plate of hot French fries:

Shelby: I can smell them. It just feels like the calories are just ready to leave the fries and come into my body and turn to fat.
Clinician: So your biggest fear is . . .
Shelby: I know it sounds crazy, but I am afraid I am going to gain 5 pounds just from sitting here with these fries.
Clinician: And how much anxiety are you experiencing on a scale of zero to 100?
Shelby: Like a 70. If I was touching them—90 or eating them 100. But even sitting here is really hard.
Clinician: So keep focusing on your anxiety and your feared outcome.

In this early stage, Shelby is being encouraged to sit with her fear of weight gain, until she learns safety and/or that she can tolerate her fear of magically absorbed calories. This exposure might be sufficient on its own to help her. However, this in vivo magical thinking exposure also might be considered as a prelude to subsequent behavioral experiments, where the exposure is accompanied by testing for any immediate effect on her weight and shape.

SUMMARY

The forms of exposure described in this chapter are all relatively experimental but fully in line with how exposure is used to treat anxiety-based disorders. They show promise with ED treatment but are in the early stages of conceptualization and development. Given their experimental nature, you will want to carefully track the degree to which the techniques are useful for individual patients and whether there are any patient characteristics that indicate who is likely to do well.

This is an area where the evidence base in EDs is quite limited, and evidence-generating practice is needed. So, we encourage you (regardless of whether you are a clinician or researcher) to add to the evidence base. As you try out and develop these methods, consider gathering sufficient data for a single-case experimental design study, case series, or even a clinical trial to help advance the clinical research base.

Summary Points—Part 3: Applying Exposure to Different Eating Disorder Problem Areas

- Exposure therapy can be applied effectively to a variety of distressing stimuli in EDs.
- Perhaps the most common type of exposure you will use with your patients is exposure to feared foods and/or eating scenarios.
- Food exposure is a helpful approach for addressing several eating-related fears, including the fear of exorbitant, uncontrollable weight gain, the fear of being powerless to prevent recurrent binge-eating episodes, and the fear of significant physical consequences (e.g., choking) related to eating (often seen in ARFID cases).
- Cue exposure involves having patients confront stimuli that elicit strong binge-eating cravings while preventing any bingeing behavior and is effective in reducing patients' binge eating and other bulimic tendencies.
- An essential component of effective exposure-based treatment for EDs involves routinely weighing the patient and openly discussing weight with them.
- Many of your patients' body image anxieties and avoidance will be effectively addressed with mirror exposure and other exposure to scenarios that are commonly avoided due to body image anxiety (e.g., wearing a swimsuit to the beach).
- Exposure can also be a useful tool in helping your patients to better cope with interpersonal and emotional stressors that often contribute to disordered eating behaviors.
- Although their scientific study is still in infant stages, there are several novel types of exposure (interoceptive, imaginal, and magical thinking exposure) that have shown promise in decreasing eating disorder symptoms.

PART 4

Important Considerations in the Delivery of Exposure

In the final section of this book, we aim to provide you with guidance around several important considerations in the delivery of exposure therapy for EDs. Specifically, we will review some important things you will need to consider when deciding whether to utilize cognitive therapy techniques in tandem with exposure. Additionally, you will learn about how those people closest to your ED patients (i.e., family and friends) can often unwittingly play a role in the maintenance and strengthening of your patients' ED symptoms, as well as how you can work with your patients' loved ones to modify their own behavior, so that they begin to "pull in the same direction" as your efforts with exposure therapy. Lastly, the final two chapters in this section describe a variety of barriers to the effective implementation of exposure therapy for EDs. Some of these barriers present themselves on a broader, organizational/institutional level, whereas others are located in the individual clinician and include clinicians' own reservations about using exposure in their practice. In addressing these clinician-level barriers, our intent is not to offend you in any way. Clinician fears about using exposure therapy are quite common. Therefore, we wanted to devote a chapter to providing you with helpful suggestions in navigating concerns you may have about using exposure in your own practice.

16

When to Use Cognitive Therapy Techniques to Enhance the Effects of Exposure

The demarcation between cognitive and behavioral strategies is much fuzzier than might appear at first glance, which makes conceptualizing the role of cognitive techniques in exposure somewhat challenging. For instance, exposure techniques arose out of behaviorism, and their initial theoretical basis came from relatively simple classical conditioning paradigms of fear acquisition and reduction. Over time, however, it became clear that fear acquisition involves cognitive processes (e.g., harm expectancies), and recent models also implicate both perceived controllability and predictability in development of fear (Hofmann, 2008; Mineka & Thomas, 1999). Similarly, as discussed in Chapter 3, understanding how exposure works has grown more complex. Although no one knows for sure exactly how exposure works, current conceptualizations of exposure processes include a prominent cognitive component (Hofmann, 2008). Indeed, as you now know, violation of harm expectancies or fear predictions is currently viewed as a critical component to successful exposure. Accordingly, it is defensible to conceptualize exposure as a cognitive therapy technique, even though its practice is, of course, behavioral in nature (Abramowitz, Deacon, & Whiteside, 2011).

On the flip side, cognitive therapy includes behavioral experiments (e.g., Beck, Rush, Shaw, & Emery, 1979) in addition to cognitive restructuring, and the line between exposure and behavioral experiments is not clear (McMillan & Lee, 2010). Indeed, the inhibitory learning model's focus on attending to harm expectancies so that they can be violated actually brings exposure closer in function to some behavioral experiments that are designed to directly test faulty appraisals (Craske, Treanor, Conway, Zbozinek, & Vervliet, 2014); hence, the characterization of exposure as just as much of a cognitive technique as it is a behavioral technique. In addition, the interacting effects of cognitions, behaviors, emotions, and physiology (e.g., the "hot cross bun" model of Padesky & Mooney, 1990) creates complexity in conceptualizing the difference between cognitive and behavioral techniques. Exposure therapy is clearly geared to modifying emotional states by reducing the use of avoidant and safety behaviors, while cognitive approaches attempt to directly address maladaptive beliefs. However, given the interaction effects in the "hot cross bun" model, you should always assume that changing one element of the system can lead to changes elsewhere. For example, the early stages of evidence-based forms of CBT for EDs have substantial effects on both anxiety and eating cognitions, despite the almost entirely exposure-based nature of the intervention at this stage (e.g., Fairburn et al., 2009; Turner, Marshall, Stopa, & Waller, 2015; Waller et al., 2018). Similarly, the use of exposure-based approaches to body image later in treatment yields cognitive changes (e.g., Key et al., 2002). Correspondingly, cognitive restructuring can, at times, yield marked changes in behavior. For instance, if your patient successfully challenges a thought that "there is nothing special about me if I am not extremely thin," he is more likely to decrease engagement in the solo pursuit of thinness and may also increase engagement with other activities and people that make him feel good about himself.

Another factor that adds clinical complexity is research from other disorders that suggests that some emotions may be more amenable to change via exposure than others. For instance, PTSD research suggests that while anxiety is highly responsive to exposure, other emotions (e.g., guilt, shame) may be better addressed via cognitive restructuring (Resick, Nishith, Weaver, Astin, & Feuer, 2002). This does not mean that other emotions never change in response to exposure. As previously noted, exposure yields changes in cognitions, which, in turn, can alter nonanxiety emotions. Nonetheless, it is important to remember that while exposure is one of the most powerful tools in your repertoire for addressing the anxiety (and disgust) components of EDs, it may not be the best tool for addressing some other emotions in some EDs patients (e.g., anger, where cognitive rehearsal can make the anger more likely to be sustained). As such, careful case conceptualization should guide your choice of tools in trying to create change with EDs.

RESEARCH GUIDANCE: BEHAVIORAL VERSUS COGNITIVE STRATEGIES

Limited research exists comparing behavioral versus cognitive strategies in the treatment of EDs. Moreover, most package treatments include both cognitive and behavioral strategies, and there have been few dismantling studies done to elucidate whether cognitive or behavioral strategies are more influential in yielding therapeutic change. There are, however, a few points you can take away from the existing empirical literature. First, although relatively few studies have reported on purely nonbehavioral approaches, existing studies tend to show a far lower level of change in ED cognitions, despite comparable samples and levels of comorbidity (e.g., Robinson et al., 2016). Second, with regard to the question of whether cognitive approaches add to the benefits of behavioral approaches to EDs, it appears that the answer differs according to the ED concerned. In a review of the literature aimed at addressing this question, Waller and Raykos (2019) concluded that cognitive-behavioral approaches are more effective than purely behavioral, exposure-based treatments for BN (e.g., Fairburn et al., 1995). Such cognitive methods include cognitive restructuring, behavioral experiments, and surveys (e.g., Fairburn, 2008; Waller et al., 2007; Waller, Turner, Tatham, Mountford, & Wade (2019). In contrast, Waller and Raykos (2019) suggest that behavioral and cognitive-behavioral approaches appear to have similar results in the treatment of AN (e.g., Channon, De Silva, Hemsley, & Perkins, 1989), indicating that cognitive elements of CBT might not add to the impact of exposure and nutrition in low-weight patients.

To summarize, the evidence to date suggests that behavioral interventions (i.e., exposure, dietary change) are more effective than cognitive methods in treating EDs and have powerful effects on cognitions as well as emotions and behaviors. However, cognitive methods can enhance exposure's effects in some EDs—particularly BN. There is no evidence that these conclusions vary with age or cognitive capacity of the patient. Clearly, however, the evidence is limited, and there is a need for more comprehensive comparisons and dismantling studies in the field (Waller & Raykos, 2019).

WHEN NOT TO USE COGNITIVE STRATEGIES: NEW ADVICE FROM THE INHIBITORY LEARNING PERSPECTIVE

Cognitive strategies have long been used in tandem with exposure to alter anxiety. For instance, early versions of CBT for panic disorder (Barlow & Craske, 1994) included use of cognitive strategies (e.g., cognitive restructuring) prior to starting interoceptive exposure and in vivo exposure. One key goal in doing so was to help panic disorder patients reduce the degree to which they engaged in catastrophizing and probability overestimation and to alter self-statements to be less threatening (e.g., "Even if I sweat during my speech, it won't be so bad" or "I have had hundreds of panic attacks and they have never killed me; I am unlikely to die during my next attack"). This brief cognitive component presumably made later exposure activities somewhat less distressing for many panic disorder patients. However, emerging evidence from the inhibitory learning model suggests that this may undercut the efficacy of exposure. More specifically, some research suggests that inhibitory safety learning is greater when the discrepancy between the harm expectancy and what happens during exposure is maximized (Craske et al., 2014). Because cognitive strategies serve to decrease this discrepancy, they may reduce the efficacy of exposure when they are used before or during exposure (Craske et al., 2014). Consider the following conversation between a clinician and a patient (Delfina), who became very avoidant of consuming any dairy products over the past year after her sister was hospitalized with a severe illness brought on by drinking spoiled milk.

Clinician: You've described your avoidance of dairy as being related to your sister's food poisoning. Please help me understand specifically what you're afraid will happen if you reintroduce dairy into your diet?

Delfina: Basically, I worry that the same thing that happened to her is going to happen to me. She got really sick from the bad milk. She was puking a lot, and she said that it felt like her insides were on fire. It sounded awful. I don't want that to happen to me.

Clinician: It certainly sounds very unpleasant. Given your belief that consuming dairy will lead to the same fate, I can understand why you avoid it. However, as we discussed last week, the continued avoidance of dairy will only strengthen your fear. If we're going to overcome this, we have to start eating dairy again. Do you remember our discussion of exposure therapy from last week?

Delfina: Yes, I remember. I know that I'll have to do the exposure with dairy so that I can hopefully get over this problem. I'm just so afraid that I'll get sick like my sister. I know it seems unlikely, but I'm still freaked out about it.

Clinician: It's clear that you're very scared of getting sick. Before we start exposure, how about we talk a little more about the likelihood that you'll actually get sick? I know that it unfortunately happened to your sister, and you're concerned it could happen to you, but what evidence is there that having dairy in your diet *wouldn't* cause you to become sick?

Delfina: Well, up until about a year ago, I had dairy regularly and never had any issues with food poisoning. I drank milk most days and ate cottage cheese regularly. I also really loved to have ice cream with my friends. None of that stuff seemed to cause any problems.

Clinician: Good. What do you think your history with dairy indicates about the safety of consuming it now?

Delfina: I suppose it means that I'm probably not going to get sick if I start to drink milk or eat cheese again.

Clinician: Excellent, Delfina. What other reasons can you think of why it's unlikely that you'll get food poisoning from dairy?

Delfina: Well, the milk that my sister drank was way past the expiration date. My sister grew up never really paying attention to those kind of things, but I'm way more careful about that stuff. I don't think I'd ever be so careless to drink milk or eat food past the expiration date.

Clinician: It sounds like you've identified plenty of reasons why the likelihood of you getting sick is very low. How about we try an exposure now to test your belief?

The clinician's use of cognitive therapy as an antecedent strategy to exposure is consistent with many manualized CBT approaches to treating anxiety disorders. However, when viewed through the lens of inhibitory learning theory, the clinician's use of cognitive therapy has inadvertently *reduced* the likely benefit that Delfina will derive from subsequent exposure activities. Given that cognitive techniques were used to diminish Delfina's fear expectancies at the outset of exposure, she will not be able to experience as substantial an expectancy violation as she would have if the cognitive strategies had never been used in the first place. On a more practical level, the clinician's use of cognitive strategies in this scenario may have been superfluous. Bear in mind that Delfina was already capable of acknowledging the low likelihood of her feared outcome even before any cognitive therapy was initiated. The clinician may have been better to simply proceed with exposure to dairy products without the pre-emptive cognitive strategies.

So what does this mean for EDs? In short, if you try to reduce your patients' anxiety prior to exposure or during exposure with either informal or formal cognitive strategies aimed at reducing their harm expectancies (e.g., changing "If I eat this piece of cake, I am going to blow up and gain 5 kilos" into "I have eaten cake before without gaining 5 kilos; eating cake is scary, but it won't add 5 kilos"), then your patients may benefit less from exposure as compared to asking them to articulate their worst fear and letting them learn that (a) it does not happen, and/or (b) they can better tolerate their distress than they expected.

WHEN TO CONSIDER COGNITIVE STRATEGIES TO AUGMENT EXPOSURE

It is beyond the scope of this chapter to consider all the ways in which cognitive techniques can be used in the treatment of EDs. Rather, we focus on conditions under which cognitive strategies may enhance the effects of exposure therapy. Note that there is almost no research to guide this advice in the area of EDs. Thus, consistent with other topics in this book, we have extrapolated based on the literature with other anxiety-based disorders, including PTSD.

When the Predominant Negative Emotion Is Not Fear

You should consider using cognitive strategies, such as cognitive restructuring, when exposure fails to alter nonanxiety cognitions and/or when the prominent emotion triggering ED behaviors is not anxiety- or disgust-based. As other authors have written extensively, in the field of anxiety and related disorders, exposure has been shown to reliably improve anxious patients' relationship with their distress (i.e., reduced anxiety duration/intensity, better anxiety tolerance). In contrast, there is limited evidence that these benefits extend to different emotional states, such as guilt, anger, and sadness (Abramowitz, Deacon, & Whiteside, 2011). Accordingly, your patients whose difficulties primarily involve nonanxiety cognitions and emotions may benefit from cognitive therapy techniques to augment exposure. Consider the following case examples of Riley and Margot.

> Riley reported a 10-year history of an ED that started after being raped by a boyfriend. Riley completed not only food and body image exposure but also imaginal and in vivo exposure (i.e., prolonged exposure; Foa & Rothbaum, 1998) to address the rape trauma. Despite marked improvement in restriction, binge eating, and purging, Riley still used binge eating and purging to manage feelings of guilt about not turning his boyfriend into campus authorities for raping him. After graduating college, Riley learned that his boyfriend had later raped at least two other people. Riley believed that the subsequent attacks were his fault. Riley's therapist used cognitive restructuring to help Riley with his beliefs that the subsequent attacks by his former boyfriend were his fault. After successful completion of cognitive restructuring, Riley became abstinent from both binge eating and vomiting.

> Margot made significant progress with her restrictive ED symptoms using exposure. However, she reported that she sometimes skipped a meal in response to her husband's treatment of her. Margot's husband often went for after-work drinks with work friends on Friday nights. Most nights he came home by 6:45 PM to eat dinner with Margot, but some nights he would call her and cancel at the last minute so he could stay out with his friends. Margot reported feeling "incensed" whenever her husband did this and noted she also responded by increasing her restriction behaviors.
>
> **Margot:** He wants me to eat and get better and then he just cancels at the last minute knowing how distressing I find that. It just makes me think—he takes me for granted. Then I look at the food I've prepared and think, "I'll get him. I won't eat, which will freak him out and then he will feel bad." Last Friday I actually threw all the food in the trash and left him a note saying that is what I had done. I then went to bed instead.
>
> Margot and her therapist used cognitive restructuring to alter her thinking about the benefits of not eating in this situation. They also used a combination of problem-solving and assertive communication skills to more directly address the husband's behavior.

Both Riley and Margot were able to derive additional benefit from the use of cognitive therapy strategies, whereas it is likely that neither would have received those benefits from exposure alone. The presence of other significant emotional disturbances outside the realm of anxiety/fear warranted an approach that more directly addressed the problematic thinking tendencies that were responsible for the maintenance of symptoms in these two patients. In our experience, properly identifying cases that warrant cognitive therapy in addition to exposure is best done through a combination of a thorough functional assessment at the outset

When Your Patient Is Extremely Hesitant to Engage

You are very likely familiar with the occurrence of a patient being hesitant to engage in exposure-based strategies. In some cases, this hesitancy and unwillingness is quite significant and is often fueled by a strong conviction that feared outcomes are bound to occur. As frustrating as this scenario can be, it is important for you to view it as an understandable response to the genuine anticipation of threat. Think about it—if you believed that doing something would almost certainly lead to an outcome that you viewed as catastrophic and/or intolerable, would you do it?

In circumstances like these, when a patient is extremely hesitant to engage with (and will likely avoid) an exposure activity, you can consider using cognitive therapy techniques to weaken your patient's belief that a catastrophic and/or intolerable outcome is imminent. Such techniques usually take the form of Socratic questioning, with the aim of helping your patient think more flexibly about the likelihood of his feared outcome. It can be particularly helpful to use open-ended questions that gently lead your patient to consider a different eventual outcome than the catastrophic one that they are dreading. This is illustrated in the following dialogue between a clinician and a patient, Meghan, who was fearful of touching any foods based on her belief that she would absorb food residue containing calories through her skin, which would lead to substantial weight gain.

> **Clinician:** Well, Meghan, I'm afraid we're in a bit of a stuck place. On the one hand, you understand how this exposure of holding a muffin in your hands could help you overcome your fear. However, we've tried to get started for the past 20 minutes, and it seems you're still unwilling to begin.
>
> **Meghan:** I know. I'm really sorry to be wasting your time. I thought I'd be able to try this, but I'm going to have to chicken out. I'm just so scared I'll wake up tomorrow and see that I've gained a massive amount of weight.
>
> **Clinician:** I understand. You described being afraid that gaining a lot of weight would mean that no one would ever love you and you'd live a life in complete isolation. I think many people would be hesitant if they believed that was a likely outcome.
>
> **Meghan:** Well, of course. Who would ever want to marry someone who looks like a huge blimp? And I just know my friends would stop returning my calls.
>
> **Clinician:** If you're willing, I'd like to discuss this idea that you can gain weight from touching food. Just how convinced are you that this is true?
>
> **Meghan:** You'll probably call me crazy, but I'm pretty convinced. Everyone has told me that it just doesn't make any sense, and I can kind of see why they say that, but it doesn't really change how I feel.

Clinician: Have you considered whether this idea pertains to other people? For example, do you believe that other people can gain weight from touching food?

Meghan: Yes, and that's why I think it's real. I never touch food, and I'm one of the smallest people in my town. I don't mean to sound critical, but it seems to me that fat people are the ones that are always around food. There is this guy who works in my office building who must weigh over 300 pounds, and he's pretty much always carrying food on him. I know that probably a lot of his weight comes from eating too much, but I also think that he could be absorbing some of the calories just from touching the food.

Clinician: I see. Let's consider some other people in your life who *don't* seem to follow this rule. Can you tell me about someone you know who touches food often and doesn't seem to gain a lot of weight?

Meghan: (*pauses to think*) Hmmm. I guess there is Gladys.

Clinician: Let's hear more about Gladys.

Meghan: Gladys is this nice girl who has an apartment on the lower level of my building. I've chatted with her a few times. She has a couple of young kids, and I always see her giving them snacks when they're playing outside. I have also seen her unwrap cupcakes and give them to her kids—iced cupcakes have a ton of calories. Come to think of it, she seems to be handling food pretty often. Just yesterday, her little girl dropped a bunch of crackers on the ground. I watched Gladys pick them up and throw them in the trash. I remember thinking I would be terrified to do that.

Clinician: So it sounds like Gladys touches food quite often. How does this seem to impact her body?

Meghan: That's the weird thing. She's really tiny.

Clinician: (*allows for silence*)

Meghan: I don't really know what to make of that. How come Gladys isn't fat by now?

Clinician: Why do think Gladys isn't fat?

Meghan: I'm not sure. It could be what other people have told me is actually true and you can't really gain weight from touching food. But I also wonder if Gladys just exercises a lot to burn the calories she absorbs. I mean, she probably chases those kids around all day.

Clinician: Let's shift gears and consider other people who probably touch food way more often than Gladys. Have you considered people who work in the food service industry?

Meghan: Not really, I guess, but I imagine most people who work in restaurants do handle food pretty often.

Clinician: Okay. Tell me what you notice about the bodies of the restaurant employees you see.

Meghan: Um, I don't ever go into restaurants. Haven't since high school. I'm too scared of them.

Clinician: (*grabs a magazine and points at the cover*) Do you know who this man is?

Meghan: Umm . . . I think he's that chef guy who yells at everyone on TV. Is his name Gordon Ramsay?

Clinician: Yes. Tell me what you know about him.

Meghan: Well, beyond his yelling, I guess I don't know that much. I think he has a lot of restaurants all over the world, so I'm assuming he touches a lot of food.

Clinician: That makes sense. Food is basically his job. Tell me what you notice about his body.

Meghan: Well, he's not fat at all. Quite the opposite. He actually has a really nice body.

Clinician: Okay, so it sounds like we've poked some holes in this idea that handling food causes massive weight gain. What are your thoughts?

Meghan: I guess I'm seeing that there are some people who maybe don't get fat from touching food. But what if they're just rare exceptions to the rule? What if I still get fat?

Clinician: I'm hoping you're in a place now where you're willing to take that risk and find out what happens. I understand you're quite afraid, but I'd really like to get going with exposure because I know it will be the best medicine for you.

Meghan: Okay, I guess I can try.

As illustrated in the previous dialogue, Meghan presented with such a challenging fixedness in her belief that cognitive therapy was needed to even get her on board with proceeding with exposure. Although we noted earlier that one risk of using cognitive strategies is that patients may not experience maximal violation of their fear expectancies, it is also important to note that patients who avoid exposure altogether experience *no* violation of their fear expectancies. Thus, in a case like Meghan's, where your patient appears genuinely on the brink of refusing exposure altogether and is possibly even at risk of dropping out of therapy, you can use cognitive therapy to help "soften" your patient's conviction in their fear expectancy such that they are willing to begin exposure.

With regard to the "dosage" of cognitive therapy that you give to your patient, the example of Meghan is a nice illustration of what we have come to call the "Goldilocks approach" to cognitive therapy. Just as Goldilocks preferred neither too much nor too little, your approach to using cognitive therapy as a precursor to exposure should aim for a "just right" amount, starting with none or very little and only adding more if it proves necessary. That is, you want to use cognitive therapy just enough to help your patient think flexibly to the extent that she is willing to subsequently engage in exposure. However, you should be careful that you are not challenging your patient's thinking to such a comprehensive extent that she approaches exposure with little doubt of a safe and tolerable outcome. Remember that your patient will benefit most from experiencing a substantial mismatch between her fear expectancy and the actual outcome she observes. You will best set the stage for this with a relatively brief period of cognitive therapy that does not result in any definitive conclusions, as Meghan's therapist did artfully.

SUMMARY

Exposure therapy is a behavioral method that has both emotional and cognitive benefits for the patient. Cognitive methods, such as cognitive restructuring, are an important weapon in your arsenal when it comes to treating EDs, but only where the exposure element is present. You should use careful functional assessment and keep in mind the exposure recommendations that follow from the inhibitory learning model when making specific decisions about when and whether to use cognitive strategies in conjunction with exposure for EDs.

17
Involving Friends, Family, and Other Loved Ones

As with many other types of psychotherapy, it often can be helpful to involve patients' friends, family members, and other loved ones in treatment (hereafter we refer to this broad constituency as family, using the term in a very inclusive way). This is especially true of exposure-based therapies, given that family members are often "part of the picture" when it comes to patients' feared stimuli, avoidance tendencies, and safety behaviors. Thus, it will behoove you to understand how you can include your patient's family members in confronting feared scenarios and stopping avoidant and safety behaviors.

It should be noted that the scope of this chapter is limited to family involvement that we have found particularly germane to exposure therapy for EDs. Although family members can play a helpful generically supportive role in the treatment, exposure therapy is predominantly an individual approach to psychotherapy. There are, of course, other therapeutic approaches that are more comprehensive in their scope of family involvement. To illustrate, FBT advocates parents and other caregivers as the primary facilitators of change in their child's eating behaviors (Lock & Le Grange, 2013). This chapter, however, is intended to provide you with a unique understanding of how family involvement can be useful in the context of exposure therapy, whatever the age of the patient.

You will need to be aware of some characteristic styles of families' responses to their loved one's avoidance and ED safety behaviors. These include accommodation/enabling and expressed emotion, both of which are associated with increased familial burden and poor treatment outcomes (described more fully in the following discussion). It will be important for you to encourage family members of your patients to stay out of these styles of interaction and instead strike a balance between empathy and firmness. Importantly, you can use sessions during which family members are present to provide coaching in effective familial involvement in exposure therapy.

THE PSYCHOSOCIAL BURDEN OF EATING DISORDERS ON FAMILIES

Before we review several characteristic patterns of how family members respond to their loved ones' ED symptoms, it is critical for you to consider the psychosocial burden that EDs create for families. Appreciating this burden will help you to understand why many families are, often out of desperation, drawn toward using unhelpful means of interacting with their afflicted loved one (i.e., your patient). Additionally, communicating your understanding of this burden to family members and providing validation of the difficult emotions they likely experience will boost their motivation to begin changing how they interact with your patients.

In short, EDs have a substantial negative impact on family functioning and well-being, whatever the age of the patient. A growing body of literature attests to the multifaceted burden that is incurred by family members of an individual with an ED. Several studies indicate that caregivers of individuals with EDs experience a high degree of emotional strain associated with trying to help their afflicted loved one (Perkins, Winn, Murray, Murphy, & Schmidt, 2004; Whitney et al., 2005; Winn, Perkins, Murray, Murphy, & Schmidt, 2004). This emotional strain contributes directly to problematic patterns of interaction between family members and the afflicted individual, which ultimately leads to the maintenance and strengthening of ED symptoms (Schmidt & Treasure, 2006). It is thus unsurprising that many caregivers of individuals with EDs endorse a host of negative effects of their caretaking experience. For example, family members report lowered quality of life (e.g., de la Rie, van Furth, De Koning, Noordenbos, & Donker, 2005) and heightened mental health problems, such as depression and anxiety disorders (Highet, Thompson, & King, 2005; Winn et al., 2007). It is worth noting that family members of individuals with OCD experience a similar nature of burden associated with their caretaking experiences (Amir, Freshman, & Foa, 2000), adding to the parallels between EDs and anxiety-based disorders.

PROBLEMATIC STYLES OF FAMILY INTERACTION

Now that you are aware of the many negative impacts that an ED often has on familial functioning and emotional well-being, we turn now to describing two characteristic patterns of familial interactions that you can expect to encounter when treating your patients—*accommodation/enabling* and *expressed emotion*. Previous research has shown that greater levels of familial burden are associated with increased engagement in these interactive styles (Whitney & Eisler, 2005; Whitney, Haigh, Weinman, & Treasure, 2007). Accordingly, when your assessment of your patient's family functioning suggests a high degree of strain, you can assume that the family is likely to be locked into one or both of these styles.

As unhelpful as these patterns of familial interaction are, it is important for you to view them as understandable efforts to cope by family members. More specifically, these ways of interacting help family members to decrease emotional tension in situations by "solving" a more tangential problem. Unfortunately, however, neither accommodation nor expressed emotion will be useful in helping your patients to overcome their ED in the shorter or longer term. Consider the following interaction at the breakfast table between Sydney, a 15-year-old girl with an ED, and her parents. In this interaction expressed emotion (i.e., father's anger) is followed by accommodation (i.e., mother's offer to make a new omelet and then agreement to change it for cereal) and then father being critical again over the costs of Sydney's ED.

Mother: Sydney, I notice you haven't touched your omelet yet. Is something the matter?

Sydney: Just look at how greasy and fatty it is! I know you probably used a whole pack of butter when you made it. No way I'm eating this.

Mother: Sydney, that's just silly. No one makes an omelet with a whole pack of butter. Please start eating.

Sydney: No! You used way too much butter. Maybe it wasn't the whole pack, but it's still too much. I'm just going to get fat if I eat this, so . . .

Father: You know what, Sydney? I can't stand one more damn argument like this. Do you have any idea what you're putting your mom and me through?

Sydney: What are you talking about?

Father: We work hard to provide everything that you need. We bend over backward to try to make you happy. Now we're both taking time away from work so that you can get treatment for your eating disorder. And this is how you thank us?

Sydney: Geez, it's not like I'm trying to have an eating disorder.

Father: Well, it doesn't look that way to me. It seems like you're just trying to get back at us for whatever reason. You doctors can say what they want about "illness," but part of me thinks you're just a spoiled brat!

Sydney: (*pauses*) Okay, fine. I'll eat the stupid omelet (*takes first bite*). Oh my gosh, I can totally taste all the butter. Gross.

Father: Is that the best you can do? How about showing a little appreciation instead of complaining all the time?

Sydney: (*sarcastically*) Gee, thanks, Mom (*takes another bite and begins to cry*).

Mother: You know, Sydney, maybe I did use a little too much butter in your omelet. Would it be better if I just made you a different one?

Sydney: Actually, it would be best if I could just have a bowl of cereal instead.

Mother: Hmmm, I don't know. Are you sure that's going to be enough?

Sydney: It'll be fine, Mom. Don't worry about it. This cereal is really filling.

Mother: Well, okay. Something is better than nothing, I suppose.

Father: Sydney, please don't throw away that omelet. Put it in the refrigerator, and I'll eat it later. I've already thrown away enough money on your eating disorder, and I'm not interested in losing any more.

Accommodation and Enabling

Accommodation occurs when your patients' family members make lifestyle, behavioral, and interpersonal choices that reduce immediate emotional strain and other pressures, but which also end up maintaining the eating problem (e.g., Sydney's mother offering to make a new omelet to calm Sydney's fears about the butter that she perceived in the original). When using accommodation, family members hope that their loved ones will believe that it is now safe to eat. However, the actual consequence is usually that your patient learns that pushing in this way results in not having to eat, and therefore your patient pushes even harder to reduce intake (e.g., Sydney declining to eat the omelet at all, persuading her mother to offer to let her eat cereal instead). In short, the family's accommodation is a short-term means of trying to defuse the tension in an ED-related situation but has the longer-term effect of maintaining or worsening the unhealthy eating patterns and interactions. Indeed, we do not know if Sydney will even eat the cereal, after all that. Note that you will sometimes see a pattern of family accommodation that relates to you, the clinician. More specifically, we find that some family members try to persuade the clinician to "go easy" on the patient and not to be so demanding of change in the short term (although they still want their loved one to recover, even if the lack of immediate change renders that implausible).

Families with higher levels of psychosocial burden associated with negative caretaking experiences are more prone to engage in accommodation of their loved one's ED. In such cases, we often see the family engaging in *enabling*. This happens when the family uses anticipatory accommodation—not even putting the patient in a position that might challenge them (e.g., never trying to go on holiday to avoid the potential of distressing Sydney about the uncontrollability of food or access to a gym). In that way, accommodation of the ED becomes a lifestyle issue (Whitney & Eisler, 2005), which means that families enable the ED to worsen by removing boundaries where challenges might occur. These behaviors parallel those seen with anxiety-based disorders. For instance, when family members agree to remove all outerwear when entering the home and don sterile overshoes so as to not distress a loved one with OCD, they are engaging in accommodation that can worsen their loved one's symptoms. Family members of people with OCD similarly may eliminate various activities (including holidays) so as to make it easier for the individual with OCD to stay in their "clean" and controllable environment. In addition, family members in both cases might aim to find a clinician for the patient who will not be challenging, to avoid ever distressing the patient.

As a result of these patterns of interaction, accommodation of the ED is associated with several negative effects. First, although giving in to the ED may decrease family members' perceived burden temporarily, it increases caregiver burden in the long run (Treasure, Gavan, Todd, & Schmidt, 2003). Additionally, given that family accommodation can be construed as a form of avoidance and/or safety behavior, it often becomes part of the ED maintenance cycle for many patients. Finally, family accommodation is correlated with reduced responsiveness to exposure therapy for anxiety-based disorders (e.g., Storch et al., 2008), and the same appears to be true in the use of exposure therapy for EDs (Anderson, Smith, Nuñez, & Farrell, 2019).

Expressed Emotion

Another problematic style of family interaction in EDs is characterized by *expressed emotion*. This can manifest in family members behaving in a critical and hostile manner, as well as being rather intrusive toward your patients (e.g., a husband calling his wife's co-workers to ensure that she ate all of her lunch). The manner in which Sydney's father interacted with her would be characterized as high in expressed emotion. Although one could certainly understand his emotional strain, his comments to her were quite critical and demeaning. It is important to note that in this example, while the father's actions were "successful" in moving Sydney toward taking a bite of the omelet, expressed emotion is not associated with long-term success in overcoming EDs. Indeed, Sydney did not end up eating the rest of the omelet, as her mother stepped in to defuse the emotional tension and her father was deflected from the task of eating by his emotional arousal. Nonetheless, the temporary success (e.g., Sydney taking a bite of omelet) is reinforcing, thereby making patterns of expressed emotion occur more frequently.

Similar to accommodation, expressed emotion is associated with a number of negative effects. For caregivers, expressed emotion is consistently linked to heightened experience of negative emotions and family dysfunction. Furthermore, high expressed emotion in the family is a reliable predictor of poorer treatment outcomes for EDs (Rienecke, Lebow, Lock, & Le Grange, 2017; Szmukler, Eisler, Russell, & Dare, 1985; Zabala, Macdonald, & Treasure, 2009). However, it is not yet clear if expressed emotion does or does not have a negative effect on treatment outcome in the context of exposure therapy for EDs.

THE MIDDLE GROUND: HELPING FAMILIES BLEND EMPATHY WITH FIRMNESS

Although the remainder of this chapter is devoted to specific ways in which family members can be successfully involved in your patients' exposure-based treatment, we first wish to offer some broad guidance for helping families navigate the difficulty of caring for their loved one without falling into the traps of accommodation/enabling or expressed emotion. The aim to this is to help the family to develop an approach based on "firm empathy" (Wilson, Fairburn, & Agras, 1997).

Like us, you will probably have had many families come to you carrying a heavy burden, desperate for relief, and feeling powerless to stop engaging in accommodation. Although many of these families acknowledge that their accommodations or patterns of expressed emotion are unhelpful, they feel unable to stop them. They feel compelled to rely on these measures due to the difficulty of tolerating their loved one's negative emotions, as well as their own fears about what would happen if they stopped accommodating (e.g., "Will my son starve?"; "Will my wife get so angry she'll leave me?"; etc.).

As a means of providing families with increased hope and motivation to change, we try to help them recognize a middle ground—between passively acquiescing to their loved one's ED rules and being overly forceful and intrusive in demanding that ED behaviors are abandoned. For many families, this middle ground involves finding an appropriate balance between empathy and firmness, such that family members can be emotionally available, validating, and encouraging of their afflicted loved one, all the while maintaining an understanding that enabling of ED-related avoidance and safety behaviors cannot continue. Being able to maintain this balance allows family members to be usefully involved in your patients' exposure activities.

THE ROLE OF FAMILY IN EXPOSURE THERAPY

We now move to describing the important role that family members can play in an exposure-based treatment approach. Although we know of no literature to date that allows for conclusions about the benefits of involving family in exposure therapy for EDs, there is a large body of literature attesting to the benefits of including family members in exposure-based treatment of OCD and related anxiety disorders (e.g., Thompson-Hollands, Edson, Tompson, & Comer, 2014). It is clear that family members can learn how to reduce accommodation behaviors in the home, while supporting their loved one in confronting feared scenarios and discontinuing safety behaviors. In the following discussion, we outline several ways that family members can become directly involved in your patients' exposure therapy.

The Family as Exposure Stimuli

One rather obvious but somewhat overlooked way that family members can be involved in treatment is to serve as exposure stimuli for their loved ones. Many ED patients report that their family members are often some of the most anxiety-evoking people to be around. Indeed, if you ask, you will find that many of your patients' fears involve eating meals as a family, wearing form-fitting clothing items in front of family members, or having physical contact (e.g., hugging) with relatives at holiday gatherings.

When family members themselves are appropriate exposure stimuli, your involvement of them in treatment becomes essential. It will be important for you to work with your patients and their families to plan exposure activities in which patients confront feared scenarios/stimuli that involve their family in some way. In doing this, you may need to direct family members to "be themselves" in the context of exposure, such that they do not attempt to censor themselves to decrease their loved one's anxiety. For example, if your patient's family have become accustomed to keeping completely silent during family meals so as to reduce your patient's distress, you need to encourage them to resume their premorbid practice of having conversation at the dinner table.

Family Members as Exposure "Coaches"

When you do not need family members to serve as exposure stimuli themselves, you can nonetheless find ways to encourage them to therapeutically increase your patient's distress during exposure. You can set this up by providing your patient's family members with instruction and ongoing guidance in serving as exposure "coaches." Perhaps one of the most effective strategies you can use in this endeavor is to encourage your patient's family to observe the manner in which you coach their loved one during exposure activities. Doing so will, among other things, allow them to see the balance between empathy and firmness that is critical to doing exposure therapy well.

Ideally, you will be able to facilitate a process whereby your patient's family members become increasingly proficient in the role of exposure coach—providing appropriate support and encouragement to their loved one, while emphasizing the need to confront fears to overcome them. This recruitment to the "team" can be especially helpful when working with patients who require some help to complete exposure homework between therapy sessions. Relatedly, caregivers of youth patients can be asked to monitor their child's successful engagement in exposure homework activities and offer reinforcement for such success (i.e., age-appropriate rewards), thus promoting continued cooperation with treatment.

Reducing and Eliminating Accommodation

As discussed earlier in this chapter, most families unfortunately fall into the trap of engaging in a number of accommodation and enabling behaviors around their loved one's ED, with negative effects for the patient (e.g., Storch et al., 2008). Reducing such accommodation over the course of exposure therapy is associated with improved treatment response (Merlo, Lehmkuhl, Geffken, & Storch, 2009).

Hence, it is crucial that you work with families of your patients to decrease their accommodation behaviors.

For some families, education is all that you will need to stop the accommodation. Many families do not recognize how their efforts to accommodate were actually countertherapeutic in the long run. Once this message registers and families can acknowledge the negative role of their accommodation in the maintenance of the ED, they typically take appropriate steps to do away with the accommodation without much guidance needed on your part. It can be useful to use a standardized measure to identify such behaviors where they are less obvious (e.g., the Accommodation and Enabling Scale for Eating Disorders; Sepulveda, Kyriacou, & Treasure, 2009). This also can be used to monitor the family's progress in reducing accommodation.

Other families will require more than just education to help them change their accommodation behaviors. This sort of circumstance warrants a careful assessment of potential factors that maintain the accommodation. Although there are many possible reasons why families continue to accommodate even after being informed about the negative effects of doing so, our clinical experience indicates that two primary factors are often involved.

- First, families have difficulty stopping accommodation because they are very *conflict-averse*. Out of fear of creating or worsening tension within the home, many families accommodate as a means to quickly circumvent situations that create conflict (e.g., Sydney's mother offering to change the food, once her husband began expressing his anger).
- Second, *distress tolerance* can play a role. Many families have great difficulty tolerating the experience of seeing their loved ones in high distress. Thus, out of their own desire to avoid the discomfort of your patient's anxious responding, many families will (albeit begrudgingly) continue to enable the ED.

Both of these maintaining factors for accommodation will require you to intervene with your patients' family members. To avoid the family feeling "accused" (and potentially responding to you in a highly defensive manner), an important first step is to communicate your understanding of their reasons for accommodation and describing the relative normalcy of this. This is similar to what you do when you explain to your patients that their safety behaviors are simultaneously understandable and problematic.

Because many family members rely on accommodating to relieve their own emotional distress, you can work with your patient's family to develop a plan in which the family will gradually decrease accommodation over the course of treatment, with the goal of eventually eliminating it. We have had success with encouraging the family to view this as their own concurrent course of exposure therapy, in which they will learn to tolerate both the patient's anxiety and their own anxiety about the patient's anxiety. Using this approach allows you to frame each exposure task with family members present as a conjoint exposure, in which both your patient and their family will confront a distressing stimulus, with the goal of violating fear expectancies. Consider our previous example of Sydney and her parents. An exposure homework task in which Sydney's parents prepare and eat a calorific meal with her could be framed as an opportunity for

- Sydney to address her food-related fears, violating expectancies of exorbitant weight gain and/or inability to tolerate anxiety, and
- Sydney's parents to confront their own anxiety about seeing her in distress (anxiety that the parents can attribute to the intervention that the therapist has introduced about not using their usual behavior patterns), violating their expectancy that they could not endure this without accommodation.

FEEDING FOR WEIGHT RECOVERY VERSUS EXPOSURE THERAPY

Elsewhere in this book we have highlighted the notion that you cannot equate feeding for weight recovery to exposure therapy because, in many cases, the conditions associated with feeding for recovery are not set up to optimally violate harm expectancies, even though some lucky patients will learn what they need to learn from this experience. Just like many clinicians, who mistakenly presume that feeding for weight recovery is equivalent to exposure therapy, many family members equate feeding for weight recovery to exposure therapy. As such, family members may be perplexed at the lack of learning that occurs during feeding for weight recovery. Further, as Murray et al. (2016) have noted, during weight recovery, patients' harm expectancies may actually be confirmed (i.e., not violated), making patients even more convinced that formerly avoided foods will, in fact, lead to rapid and potentially never-ending weight gain.

Just as you can use psychoeducation to teach patients about exposure therapy, you also can teach family members. In particular, it can be helpful to teach family members that exposure works best when harm expectancies are clearly violated and that exposure should be mixed up to the greatest degree possible to enhance safety learning. Indeed, Murray et al. (2016) provide case study evidence that parents can be taught to guide adolescent children in clearly identifying harm expectancies and then carefully tracking evidence that falsifies those expectancies, even after harm expectancies were initially confirmed by refeeding. In summary, be prepared to use psychoeducation to educate family members about some of the theory of the inhibitory learning model, so that they understand how to optimally serve as exposure coaches.

SUMMARY

Although exposure-based treatments are most commonly implemented in an individual therapy format, involving families in exposure can boost the likelihood of a successful treatment outcome. Many families will need your instruction and careful guidance in sidestepping the common pitfalls of accommodating their loved one's ED symptoms and/or engaging in patterns of highly emotionally charged and critical responding toward their loved one (i.e., expressed emotion). You have several useful options to involve family members directly in your patients' exposure activities. Utilizing these options effectively will help to instill a collective "exposure mindset," in which the family are all on the same page in confronting anxiety-evoking stimuli and eliminating use of safety behaviors.

18

Addressing the Impact of Different Settings and Institutional Resistance

In Chapter 19, you will be introduced to the intra-individual factors that contribute to individual clinicians failing to implement exposure in an effective way (or at all). However, it is equally important to understand how the clinical system that you work in can impair your ability to make the best use of exposure therapy for EDs. Thus, you may need to address systemic barriers in your clinical setting—we refer to this as "institutional resistance"—before you are even able to undertake effective exposure therapy with your patients.

Addressing institutional resistance can be tricky. You may need to alter team dynamics, challenge clinic protocols (both explicit and implicit), and push for changes in service provision and shared practice. To help you understand some of the types of institutional resistance you may face, we have drawn upon our collective experience of encountering such resistance and selected several of the more extreme (and annoying) examples to present. Although some of the examples we provide may seem to border on absurd, each of our examples is a genuine one.

WAYS THAT TEAM DYNAMICS CAN INTERFERE WITH USE OF EXPOSURE THERAPY

ED treatment often, although not always, involves a treatment team. Thus, a key issue in the delivery of evidence-based treatments for EDs is whether a given team shares common goals and philosophies or whether individual members differ in what they see as achievable and how to go about it. Where there are differences, you will likely see team dynamics that reduce the feasibility and effectiveness of exposure therapy.

Exposure is a technique that may particularly engender disparate attitudes among team members. Exposure is embraced by many therapists who treat anxiety-based disorders both because of the empirical evidence that it works and because they personally have seen the tremendous benefit many patients experience. However, other therapists (who typically have less training in exposure) view exposure as "mean." Indeed, in a *New York Times* editorial about exposure for adult anxiety disorders, which was titled "The Cruelest Cure," some therapists reportedly described exposure as "torture, plain and simple" (Slater, 2003). Further, in case you think we are being excessive in warning you about colleagues who may themselves find exposure anxiety-provoking, consider this quote from a therapist in the same editorial: "Just hearing about [exposure] gives me the fight-or-flight response." In summary, if you work in a team-based setting and you want to maximize the benefit of exposure, be prepared to possibly encounter the following issues within your team.

Team Members Try to Protect the Patient From the "Nasty" Exposure Therapist

Despite evidence from both efficacy and effectiveness studies that recovery from EDs (a) is possible and (b) requires patients to face their fears, many clinicians assume that patients are fragile and rarely recover fully (or at all). As a result, if you work with a team-based approach and want to implement exposure, you may find yourself at odds with some (or even all) of the members of your team. Although *you* know that exposure can help your patients, even though it initially raises anxiety, your risk-averse colleagues may only focus on the short-term increase in your patients' anxiety, which they presume is bad. As a result, members of your team may argue with you about the use of exposure, particularly as indicated by the inhibitory learning model. If your primary aim is to keep a peaceful team dynamic, you may find yourself having to make compromises that either weaken the exposure work or lead you to abandon it altogether. Examples that we have encountered include the following:

- The team agrees to let the clinician undertake exposure, but only in tiny steps, rather than in a way that could produce stronger and sustained benefits (e.g., "Just aim for very small changes in eating, or your patient might complain and then we will have lots of paperwork to do").
- A team member insists on offering patients medication to "calm them down" when they are due to have their exposure sessions.
- The team labels the exposure therapist "Miss Nasty" in a jokey fashion with the aim of applying social pressure to get the that therapist to change course.
- The team tells patients that they will place another member of staff outside the therapy room so that patients can run off and get comforted if they get too scared by "Miss Nasty" in the session.
- An inpatient team decides to reduce weight targets for an AN patient to avoid the team's concerns that the patient will experience short-term

anxiety about faster weight gain and will feel that the team does not care about her as a result. In these types of cases, we have seen patients effectively be allowed to stay at a very low weight or even negotiate for *lower* weights than at admission, with the team accepting this in the (forlorn) hope that patients will bond with the team and turn around to make clinical progress.
- The team (whether knowingly or unknowingly) undermines the intensity of exposure by concurrently encouraging frequent practice of anxiety reduction strategies, such as diaphragmatic breathing or progressive muscle relaxation.
- The team tries to distract the patient at meals with conversation or stories so as to reduce anxiety generated by eating feared foods.

In short, when your team is risk-averse and focuses on short-term anxiety (rather than long-term maintenance of the ED) as the primary risk, team dynamics can become a problem that you will need to address explicitly with your team.

Rules About How the Eating Disorder Team Operates Can Impair Exposure

Team-based operational rules are usually put in place to avoid confusion and ensure that the range of necessary therapeutic tasks actually occur (e.g., rules about who will prescribe any medication; who provides dietary advice; who delivers the therapy). Such rules optimally should be set up or adapted with the primary aim of maximizing effective therapeutic interventions. Unfortunately, this point is sometimes lost, as it is treated as secondary to a desire to keep the rules in place so that no clinician feels that their role is being undermined and so that the team does not need to navigate new and less charted waters.

A classic example of such thinking frequently occurs in the weighing of patients. As noted in Chapter 12, you personally need to weigh your patient during CBT and in other evidence-based therapies (Waller & Mountford, 2015). In CBT, the maximum expectancy violation is achieved by weighing the patient at the point in the session when they are most anxious about their weight—in other words, immediately after you have discussed the patient's food intake over the previous week. That timing means that the patient's anxiety is at a peak ("I ate *so* much"), and they are likely to believe that their weight will have gone up by a very large amount—an expectancy that is violated by their weight being shown to have moved little or not at all (Waller, Turner, Tatham, Mountford, & Wade, 2019).

Yet, in many settings, other team members will resist this because they view weighing as "my job." For example, imagine that you are a therapist using CBT and your team rule is that the dietitian weighs all patients every week to ensure patients' safety. Note that this is not a problem from an exposure perspective as long as you can *also* weigh your patient as part of exposure and CBT (Waller

& Mountford, 2015). However, it *is* a major problem if you are not allowed to weigh your patient because the team does not want the dietitian to appear redundant or untrusted. In deciding to spare the feelings of a colleague and follow the "rules," your team undermines therapeutic effectiveness and prevents your patient making a necessary link between eating and weight. Further, as noted earlier, weighing in different contexts (you and the dietitian create different contexts) can enhances safety learning. Therefore, preventing these two weighing opportunities can have the negative effect of inhibiting the patient's learning that anxiety over weighing is not necessary.

In such circumstances, for your patients' benefit, it will be important for you to push your team to review, and likely change, its "nonnegotiables" about how the team needs to work. Other examples of these nonnegotiables include rules about who manages dietary intake or monitors physical conditions. They might also include rules about the degree to which meals can be flexible and even rules that ban having different rules for different patients. Note that even considering such changes might be concerning to some team members. Yet, the principles of exposure can apply here too. Encourage your team to embrace a more flexible mindset and try changing. This will give everyone a chance to see whether expectancies are confirmed or violated and whether all of you can "roll" with change better than you had assumed you could.

The Team Is Only as Strong as Its Weakest Link

It is worth noting that your patients often can be relied on to tell you who are the "weakest links" in a team either verbally (e.g., some patients will just disclose without prompting that a particular clinician helps them escape their anxiety) or through their behaviors (e.g., you notice that your patient prefers eating with the "nice" staff person who tries to distract patients during meals). In some cases, the weak links will expose themselves without assistance from your patients. As an example, in one inpatient service, the patients were reviewed regularly for progress. A lack of adequate weight gain understandably resulted in the team prescribing greater intake of food, and this was conveyed to the patient. However, once the patient left the room and the team meeting ended, the "weak link" team members would each go to a particularly powerful team member to explain to him that the planned food intake was unreasonable and would wreck the fragile therapeutic alliance. They would then ask him to petition the remainder of team members to reduce that food prescription. Within minutes, the powerful team member would call a second review meeting and make that request. It took several weeks before the "strong link" team members identified this pattern. Unfortunately, they took even longer before they challenged the powerful team member about this, for fear of upsetting that team member. Sadly, team dynamics can end up being prioritized over the needs of patients if we do not address problems at a systemic level.

As you already know, use of exposure will elicit anxiety in your ED patients—indeed, such anxiety is a requirement for successful exposure. However, exposure also can evoke anxiety among other members of your clinical team, and one common fear is that exposure will impair the therapeutic alliance, even though research suggests that exposure does not harm the therapeutic relationship (e.g., Kendall et al., 2009). In these circumstances, it is critical that such disparities in perception are identified and discussed openly, so that your team as a whole can identify its own avoidant and safety behaviors and reduce them by accepting short-term team anxiety to maximize benefits for your patients. In short, the team needs to work on a common philosophy of "firm empathy" (Wilson, Fairburn, & Agras, 1997) that we have referred to previously in this book. This will require you to identify the weak link clinicians whose emphasis on other aspects of treatment (especially the working alliance) is counterproductive. You will then need to engage them in the firm element of that stance, so that the team works with a common goal.

COMMON SERVICE-LEVEL ISSUES IN THE DELIVERY OF EXPOSURE THERAPY FOR EATING DISORDERS

While the nature of EDs means that we should consider applying exposure therapy in many contexts, services sometimes have rules and structures that interfere with best clinical practice and reduce your chances of getting the best possible outcome for your patients. Some of these are very obvious, particularly when considering outpatient settings. However, more intensive clinical services also can have a range of very profound service-level issues that your team will need to consider. The common theme of all of the issues raised in this section is that you cannot address them as an individual clinician—you will need to engage your clinical team and managers in systems-level change based around patients' needs for the most effective therapy possible.

Outpatient Service Issues

Given the previously outlined team issues, it might appear that outpatient services are where it should be easiest to deliver exposure therapy to ED patients, as outpatient clinicians typically have far more independence to do so. However, this is not always the case, as service constraints can apply here. Indeed, service rules can present a big enough barrier that you will need to directly address them with administrators and/or other clinicians to facilitate the delivery of exposure to your patients. Common real-life examples that you may encounter include services that:

- Do not have basic equipment, such as weighing scales in each therapy room, or do not calibrate those scales to ensure that the findings are reliable if the clinician has to use different rooms at different times.
- Do not allow clinicians to weigh the patient or encourage blind-weighing, where the patient is not told their weight (e.g., Forbush, Richardson, & Bohrer, 2015).
- Have rules about staff behavior that make the environment unrepresentative of everyday life (e.g., rules about staff not eating anywhere that patients might see them).
- Do not have mirrors or do not allow mirrors anywhere that patients might see themselves, thus preventing the use of mirror exposure and facilitating avoidance of mirrors.
- Prohibit staff from undertaking field work with the patient (e.g., going out of the clinic to identify feared foods in a local market; requiring risk assessments because you are planning to do something that is not usual).

We have seen these issues in many outpatient services, including some very prominent services with substantial national and international reputations. While some of these issues are also present in more intensive care settings, they are likely to be more noteworthy in outpatient settings, and they may be the only thing that prevents you from implementing exposure therapy. Again, the key is to work on these as a team, rather than on your own.

Intensive Eating Disorder Care Settings

Eating is a fear-inducing experience for your patients. Yet, some environments have the potential to either enhance and maintain fear or artificially dampen it, particularly in services that involve working more intensively (e.g., inpatients or day patients). Thus, you will need to understand the nature of the clinical setting and how that interacts with the team's own propensity for avoidance and safety behaviors.

TEAM SAFETY BEHAVIORS

Intensive ED care settings (e.g., in-patient; day-patient) can reduce or enhance patients' fear, depending on how they organize the eating and nutrition elements of their programs. Often, services engage in team-level safety behaviors. Difficulties arise when such services aim for:

- Rigidity of diet (e.g., "Potatoes must weigh exactly 200 grams, and if they do not, then we will slice bits off until they do");
- Predictability of intake (e.g., "Everyone must order their choices 2 days in advance so they know what to expect and we have an easier time planning");

Addressing the Impact of Different Settings

- Lack of personalization (e.g., "Everyone must eat the same thing, to prevent envy and disputes"); and
- Continuity (e.g., "Uninterrupted weight gain is the only acceptable target").

Each of these rules can be seen as a codified safety behavior on the part of the clinical team members, in so much as the rules avoid the risk of being viewed as not doing their jobs properly and decrease anxiety about potential challenges caused by flexibility and variability. However, each of these rules results in restricting the range of exposure experiences, thus reducing the amount of inhibitory learning that patients can achieve. This means that recovery is less likely to be achieved or generalized, regardless of weight gain in the short term.

Impact of Intensive Care Settings on Patient Safety Behaviors

Of course, it is not only clinicians who undertake safety behaviors to reduce their anxiety in these intensive care settings. In fact, we more typically associate this pattern with those experiencing EDs. Patients in intensive care settings are often extremely underweight and already experience profound fear of eating and food. Further, when patients lack control over whether they are going to eat or how much, that anxiety is only exacerbated. Therefore, the remaining option that your patients will identify is to use avoidance and safety behaviors to reduce the ingestion or retention of the food. Some such behaviors are relatively well-known and controlled for (although rarely with exposure in mind), including the rule that many services have about patients not being allowed to visit the bathroom or exercise for an hour after eating.

However, your patients' anxiety-reducing behaviors in such settings will be far more diverse than such simple efforts. If you work in such a context, you will know the efforts that many patients make to avoid food or its feared impact on weight before, during, and after eating. These include (but are not limited to):

- Day patients who arrive too late or leave too early to be fully monitored in their eating;
- Patients who induce or feign illness to avoid eating;
- Patients who exercise subtly while at the table (e.g., "restless legs");
- Patients who move their food around or make it inedible; and
- Individuals who secrete food by adding it to potted plants, smearing it on the underside of the table, hiding it in their pockets or undergarments, or even smearing it in their hair to conceal it.

While such patients are often described as being "devious" or "difficult," you should beware of accepting such a viewpoint. These patients are extremely anxious and are often doing the only thing that they can think of to reduce their anxiety in the short term.

Of course, as with any other avoidance and safety behaviors, you need to consider the longer-term consequences. A patient in such a setting who fails to gain weight is likely to be observed more intensively, which will make it harder and harder to prevent weight gain and make the environment more and more rigid in how it handles mealtimes and snacks. This pattern will add to your patient's sense of vulnerability and increase their anxiety, so that any resultant, unavoidable weight gain will be experienced as completely out of control. Furthermore, the rigidity of the eating setting and rules means that your patient (a) will likely experience treatment as involuntary and (b) has little or no chance of generalizing their change in eating to other settings, foods, etc. Therefore, upon discharge to a completely different context (e.g., outpatient clinic, home) your patient will simply have no resources to successfully manage their anxiety, because their very limited and narrow, context-dependent inhibitory learning will not generalize beyond the intensive care setting. In summary, we should not be surprised at the high relapse rates when patients leave intensive care settings.

USING FOOD AND EATING EXPOSURE IN INTENSIVE CARE SETTINGS

Given this summary, you should consider the principles of inhibitory learning when planning dietary change for your patients in such settings. Once the core issue of biological safety has been addressed and you have oriented your patient to the rationale for exposure, the most effective long-term approach to dietary change is likely to be based on low levels of predictability and high levels of diversity (e.g., "What fast-food place shall we go to today?"). It will also be individualized (e.g., "Peter needs to learn that weight gain is controllable before moving on to day-patient care, so we need to reduce his diet so that he stays stable in weight for the next 2 weeks. This means we will have to tolerate the other patients complaining to us that he is being treated as special and explain to them why this is what we are doing right now for him"). This overall approach will be harder for the team to impose because it involves more uncertainty for us. Yet we cannot be good exposure therapists and avoid this uncertainty. Greater ability to design exposure tasks that let individual patients learn what they need to know is simply too important if the goal is to instill robust, generalizable safety learning.

SUMMARY

There is a level of institutional resistance to the implementation of evidence-based therapies—particularly exposure therapy. This can manifest in the team dynamic (e.g., the team that treats the exposure therapist as a threat to the patient's equanimity), in outpatient service provision issues, and particularly in more intensive care provision issues. In all of these, the context in which patients are exposed to eating needs to be appropriately diverse to ensure that they are able to voluntarily engage in exposure therapy around eating and overcome their use of avoidance and safety behaviors in the broader context of everyday life. Yet, the team and service can purposefully or inadvertently enhance the patient's use of avoidance and safety behaviors if the structures are not well thought out and responsive to patients' needs. These need to be addressed by the team as a whole, rather than by the individual clinician, if the maximum benefit for the patients is to be realized when implementing exposure therapy.

Thus far, we have only considered implementation issues that relate to the service. It is just as important (if not more so) to consider the individual clinician's contribution to the success or failure of exposure therapy. The next chapter will address what you can do to ensure that you are maximally effective in delivering exposure therapy to your patients.

19
Dealing With Clinicians' Fears About Using Exposure

It is clear that exposure is a highly useful tool in the treatment of EDs. Nonetheless, you will encounter numerous challenges in maximizing the benefit of exposure for your patients. The previous chapter outlined situational and institutional factors that can impact your use of exposure in everyday practice. However, while addressing those social and environmental factors will improve your ability to use exposure, you also need to consider the impact of another factor—namely, clinicians themselves. When you or your supervisee are helping your patients to address their ED behaviors, you need to consider what you bring into the room with you that might facilitate or hamper the effective use of exposure.

GENERAL CLINICIAN FACTORS UNDERPINNING OUR FAILURE TO USE EVIDENCE-BASED APPROACHES

In this chapter, we will discuss evidence that indicates that clinicians' own characteristics influence the use of CBT skills, with a particular emphasis on exposure. This concept of clinician factors is addressed within the broader construct of "therapist drift" (e.g., Waller, 2009), although indications that clinician factors are a problem date back much further. In particular, Meehl (1954, 1973, 1986) highlighted the following interlinked phenomena decades ago:

- *Reliance on clinical judgment rather than evidence-based practice*
  Clinicians tend to value their clinical judgement more than the research, even though the evidence says that we should focus on the research to get the best outcomes for our patients overall (e.g., Meehl, 1954; Grove, Zald, Lebow, Snitz, & Nelson, 2000). Unfortunately, becoming a clinician does not save you from the cognitive biases associated with all human thinking, Therefore, clinical judgement is subject to a range of reasoning problems (e.g., confirmation bias, the availability heuristic). In contrast, research methodology is designed

to systematically reduce such biases. The overvaluing of clinical judgement is likely to be the reason that so few clinicians routinely use treatment manuals to guide their work (e.g., Addis & Krasnow, 2000; Waller, Mountford, et al., 2013), even though their use is associated with better outcomes (e.g., Addis & Waltz, 2002; Cukrowicz et al., 2011).

- *The "spun glass theory of the mind"*
  Meehl (1973) used this construct to describe how some clinicians act in a way that shows that they see their patients as "fragile" (like a spun-glass Christmas tree bauble). Unfortunately, little has changed in the decades since Meehl made this observation. Consider this quote from Slater (2003) by a psychiatrist at a major medical center: "I think very few patients can tolerate that adrenaline-based approach." This perception results in clinicians failing to push their patients to change in therapy sessions, for fear of "breaking" them. These clinicians back off from asking patients to change, resulting in a reciprocal cycle of avoidance between clinicians and their patients. This pattern means that neither feels anxious in the short term, but the therapy has little chance of success (e.g., Waller & Turner, 2016). It can be argued that the same occurs in supervision sessions, whenever supervisors back off from pushing clinicians to change their therapy behavior.

- *The "broken leg exception"*
  Meehl (1954) identified how clinicians regularly treat individual patients as exceptions to the rules of what works in therapy, usually for reasons that are not valid (e.g., "I cannot use exposure with this patient—she has comorbid depression/he uses alcohol/she is female/he is too old, etc."). This is a well-established feature of clinical work with anxiety (e.g., Deacon, Farrell, et al., 2013; Meyer, Farrell, Kemp, Blakey, & Deacon, 2014), but occurs in most psychotherapeutic practice.

Given these phenomena, you will see that it is very easy for clinicians to feel as though they can and should excuse their patients from undertaking a relatively "firm" approach such as exposure, which intentionally raises patient anxiety. In short, many clinicians worry that asking their patients to undertake exposure will distress and/or damage their patients, make their patients leave therapy because of a ruptured therapeutic alliance, or even result in a complaint (despite the lack of support for any of these outcomes; e.g., Deacon & Farrell, 2013; Olatunji, Deacon, & Abramowitz, 2009; Kendall et al., 2009). Consequently, clinicians use their clinical judgement to conclude that the specific patient or even whole groups of patients should be excluded from exposure therapy (e.g., "My patient is not psychologically minded enough"; "My patients are just too complex for the evidence to apply"), even though that judgment is less effective (and more likely to be flawed due to normal human reasoning biases) than relying on the research evidence about what works (Grove et al., 2000).

CLINICIAN FACTORS THAT INFLUENCE THE USE OF EXPOSURE IN ANXIETY DISORDERS

There is clear evidence that many clinicians do not apply exposure therapy at all or appropriately to a range of anxiety-based disorders (e.g., Hipol & Deacon, 2013). For example, imaginal exposure is not commonly used in the treatment of PTSD despite clear empirical evidence of its value (e.g., van Minnen, Hendricks, & Olff, 2010). In some cases, clinicians are unaware of core exposure methods, but others choose not to use them when they could. For example, even when clinicians are aware of exposure-based approaches to PTSD, many report feeling uncomfortable about using them (Becker, Zayfert, & Anderson, 2004), despite the fact that potential patients do not have the same reservations (Becker et al., 2009). Similarly, exposure-based methods are underutilized in OCD (Stobie, Taylor, Quigley, Ewing, & Salkovskis, 2007). Given the extensive empirical support for exposure in the treatment of these and other disorders, we must all ask: Why does this happen?

You will likely not be surprised to hear that clinicians' *negative beliefs about exposure* clearly play a role in whether and how we apply exposure therapy (e.g., Deacon, Farrell et al., 2013; Deacon, Lickel, Farrell, Kemp, & Hipol, 2013; Farrell, Deacon, Kemp, et al., 2013; Whiteside, Deacon, Benito, & Stewart, 2016). Indeed, negative beliefs about exposure for anxiety disorders transcend geographical boundaries, existing in multiple parts of the world (e.g., Farrell, Deacon, Kemp, et al., 2013; Pittig, Kotter, & Hoyer, 2019). Just as important are our own *anxiety* levels. Multiple studies using physiological indices of distress have shown that clinicians are as anxious during exposure therapy as their patients are (Schumacher et al., 2014, 2015). Further, Harned, Dimeff, Woodcock, & Contrera (2013), Meyer et al. (2014), and Parker and Waller (2017) have all shown that clinicians' own anxiety is associated with poorer uptake and use of exposure for anxiety disorders. Thus, it is clear that some of us are more likely to exclude our patients from exposure therapy for reasons that have to do with our own (vs. patient) characteristics. This conclusion is supported by the fact that biological indicators of clinician anxiety (particularly skin conductance response) are associated with whether clinicians choose to offer patients exposure therapy (Levita, Salas Duhne, Girling, & Waller, 2016).

In short, as Meehl (1986) has pointed out, by virtue of being human, clinicians tend to use a number of heuristics (i.e., mental shortcuts) that influence our nonuse of evidence-based treatments. These "rules of thumb" apply particularly strongly to our failure to use exposure for anxiety disorders. In particular, we are less likely to use exposure if we hold negative beliefs about it and if we have higher levels of trait anxiety. This leads us to an important question—namely, does this evidence translate to how we treat EDs?

CLINICIAN FACTORS THAT INFLUENCE THE USE OF EXPOSURE FOR EATING DISORDERS

Considering the specific case of EDs, the findings on clinicians' use of exposure appear very similar to those for anxiety disorders:

- Clinicians routinely omit exposure-based methods when delivering CBT for EDs (e.g., Mulkens, de Vos, de Graaff, & Walle, 2018; Waller, Stringer, & Meyer, 2012).
- Clinicians' positive beliefs about the value of the therapeutic alliance are associated with a lower use of the key exposure element of changing eating patterns (D'Souza Walsh, Davies, Pluckwell, Huffinley, & Waller, 2019). Stronger beliefs about the value of the therapeutic alliance in CBT also are associated with less use of exposure-based methods, including weighing and structured eating (Mulkens et al., 2018).
- Clinician anxiety results in poorer application of exposure-based methods in CBT for EDs (e.g., Mulkens et al, 2018; Turner, Tatham, Lant, Mountford, & Waller, 2014).

Other factors also influence our use of exposure for EDs. In particular, ED clinicians who are younger are less likely to use exposure (Turner et al., 2014), which runs contrary to the anxiety field, where younger clinicians are *more* likely to use exposure (Deacon, Farrell, et al., 2013). One key difference between EDs and anxiety disorders may explain this. ED patients are notoriously more ambivalent about treatment than anxiety disorder patients. Thus, ED clinicians may need more time to become more willing to use "tougher" methods with ED patients and to lose some of that "spun-glass theory of the mind." It also could be argued that we begin our careers as ED clinicians focusing more on empathy rather than the ever-important balance of firmness and empathy (Wilson, Fairburn, & Agras, 1997). That is an issue for our likely clinical effectiveness. If those of us who work with EDs view the alliance and core therapy techniques (including exposure) as alternative therapeutic strategies, rather than complementary ones (D'Souza Walsh et al., 2019), we will impair the impact of existing evidence-based treatments. Younger clinicians might be more prone to such conflictual stances.

To summarize, our characteristics as clinicians have the potential to interfere with therapy by making us less likely to deliver exposure-based methods for EDs. This is largely the same pattern as found with anxiety disorders, which suggests that we can draw lessons from the field of anxiety as to how to enhance our use of exposure for ED patients.

ENCOURAGING CLINICIANS TO USE EXPOSURE FOR EATING DISORDERS

Several theory- and evidence-based methods have been implemented to enhance clinician use of exposure in the field of anxiety disorders. Some of these have been extended to work with ED clinicians, but others still need evidence to support their use with this clinical group. Although research suggests that some types of clinicians may be more or less likely to use exposure (see previous discussion), we do not focus on that here—because we are *all* susceptible to the biases of clinical judgment. Further, while some of us may be less anxiety prone as clinicians (and thus more likely to use exposure), virtually all exposure therapists will feel the urge to avoid exposure at some point in our careers—it is pretty much inevitable. Thus, we should all assume that we can always improve.

Increasing Clinician Knowledge

A key issue here is that clinicians often lack knowledge and understanding of exposure therapy, as Becker et al. (2004) found among clinicians working with PTSD. In the field of EDs, probably the more obvious example of this deficit is the lack of knowledge of the inhibitory learning approach—it took almost a decade to make the transfer from the field of anxiety disorders into the ED literature (e.g., Murray et al., 2016; Reilly, Anderson, Gorrell, Schaumberg, & Anderson, 2017; Waller et al., 2019). However, the time taken to get evidence into general clinical practice (15–20 years; Institutes of Medicine, 2001) cannot fully explain lack of awareness when treatments have been known for a very long time (e.g., Becker et al., 2004). Training courses and continuing professional development need to ensure that clinicians are aware of the basics and core therapy techniques—not just novel approaches. As clinicians, we need to open those foundational books, rather than letting them sit on our shelves.

Changing Clinician Beliefs and Attitudes About Exposure

Different methods have been proposed for addressing clinicians' negative attitudes regarding exposure. These include dissonance-based approaches (e.g., asking clinicians to make the case for exposure) and the use of case examples (Farrell, Deacon, et al., 2013). Fortunately, the evidence does suggest that we can change clinician beliefs and attitudes about exposure for anxiety disorders using a didactic or workshop approach to educate clinicians (Deacon, Farrell et al., 2013). The same holds true of teaching sessions for clinicians working with EDs (Waller, D'Souza Walsh & Wright, 2016), which result in the same substantial level of change. Importantly, the effects for ED clinicians were greater if they had poorer attitudes at the outset of the training, suggesting that those who are least likely to use exposure therapy are the most likely to experience positive change in attitudes to exposure for EDs. In summary, the evidence shows that clinicians' negative attitudes to exposure can be changed using case-based education.

Reducing Clinician Anxiety

Clearly, given its role in the non-delivery of exposure therapy for EDs, it is important to consider how we can reduce clinician anxiety about exposure therapy. It is possible that some clinicians are "born" exposure therapists, due to having higher trait cognitive and biological levels of tolerance of uncertainty (e.g., Levita et al., 2016). However, if you find that exposure makes you anxious, you should not give up—after all, we know that we can reduce anxiety in patients, so why not in clinicians? Moreover, it is likely that many of the (albeit limited group of) clinicians who seem to take to exposure like "ducks to water" do so because they have previously had successful experiences with exposure elsewhere in their lives.

One of the best ways to become less anxious about exposure, and to gain greater confidence in its efficacy, is to experience the benefits of exposure first hand by facing your own fears and deliberately invoking anxiety. Try riding the same roller coaster many times in a row and experience not only the loss of anxiety (or what some call the "rush") as well as the loss of sensations. This is analogous to interoceptive exposure, and is actually a bit sad for those of us who actually like roller coasters and their associated physical sensations. Fearful of horses, swimming, motorcycle riding, or scuba diving? Take lessons. Teachers of these skills are typically quite good layperson exposure therapists, as they have to help frightened learners overcome fear all the time.

Further, if you have a clinically significant (or even sub-clinical) anxiety disorder, enter treatment with an experienced exposure therapist. Learning to overcome your own anxiety is a critical component of conducting exposure therapy because, as noted above, exposure makes all of us anxious at some point. Overcoming your own anxiety as a clinician is easier if you adopt the exposure lifestyle we encouraged you to promote to your patients.

Farrell, Deacon, Dixon and Lickel (2013) also have suggested that we should use "exposure for exposure therapists"—namely, offer simulated exposure therapy exercises to reduce clinician anxiety. A preliminary test utilizing such an approach showed promising results in reducing clinician negative beliefs and anxiety about exposure and consequently improving the quality of exposure therapy delivery (Farrell, Kemp, Blakey, Meyer, & Deacon, 2016). While promising, this approach requires further evidence, before it can be advocated further and extrapolated to the ED field. So in the meantime, practice facing your own fears in your daily life.

Changing Clinician Behaviors

One key area where we need to consider clinicians' own behaviors is in the area of eating itself. For example, when considering the approach to interpersonal exposure that Vitousek (2019) suggests (see Chapter 14), it is clear that we need to be comfortable with eating normally (or even unusually) to facilitate exposure for our patients. This is also a necessary skill for some OCD clinicians, whose patients will avoid food for fear of contamination. You cannot ask your patient to eat a food contaminated by wiping it on the ground if you are not willing to also eat the contaminated food. In summary, exposure often requires modeling the very eating behavior that you want your patient to adopt.

However, what if you are a picky eater or have a more substantial history of an ED? We firmly believe that clinicians who have had eating problems in the past can function successfully as clinicians for EDs post their own recovery. Indeed, there is evidence that patients find disclosures of such a history helpful if they are handled well (e.g., Wasil, Venturo-Conerly, Shingleton, & Weisz, 2019). However, self-defined recovery is highly variable, and we should be attentive to the possibility that some of us will indeed struggle to implement exposure as Vitousek (2019) suggests (e.g., eat a big, extravagant dessert while your patient eats a small bowl of ice cream). If you find it challenging to eat in this way, again consider exploring the value of exposure in your own life, this time focused around food. Similarly, if you are supervising other clinicians in treating EDs, be aware that this is an issue that requires consideration in supervision.

In terms of changing clinician eating behavior, you can consider methods that are effective in changing other health-related behaviors, such as implementation intentions (e.g., Toli, Webb, & Hardy, 2016). However, it remains likely that the most effective way of getting clinicians to undertake and see the value of exposure therapy for EDs is to get them to undertake exposure therapy (in this case to food) and to learn from the experience and the outcomes. Again, supervision is going to be key in any such change of clinician behavior and development of skills.

Supervision

In principle, supervision should make us better exposure therapists, by addressing the previously raised points. Becoming a supervisor should encourage us to enhance our knowledge, modify our attitudes, increase our tolerance of uncertainty, and change our behaviors. Supervision also should address all of these issues for trainees, both directly and through management of the trainee professional development. For example, it could be argued that clinicians-in-training should first focus on ensuring that their exposure skills are up to scratch before undertaking further training in other techniques that might be less effective or that could clash with the effectiveness of exposure therapy for EDs.

However, there are important caveats that we, as supervisors, should all consider with regards to our skills and the outcomes for patients:

1. As supervisors, we may not be very good at judging the skills of our supervisees. For instance, Dennhag, Gibbons, Barber, Gallop, and Crits-Christoph (2012) found that supervisors rate their supervisees' CBT skills consistently more positively than independent judges. This overestimation is similar to the finding that we, as clinicians, consistently overestimate our own skills and patient outcomes (e.g., Walfish, McAlister, O'Donnel, & Lambert, 2012).
2. Supervision models are relatively inconsistent, and most have little or no focus on the outcome for patients (Simpson-Southward, Waller, & Hardy, et al., 2017).
3. At least in the field of depression, supervisors respond to anxious clinicians by focusing less on therapeutic techniques, but only if the clinician is female (Simpson-Southward et al., 2016). This pattern occurs regardless of the gender of the supervisor.

In short, while supervision has the potential to encourage all of the clinical development and monitoring that are needed to create effective exposure therapists, we need to be aware of the ways in which supervision can also be prone to "drift." Thus, we need to focus supervision of exposure therapists on clinical outcomes and progress. We also need to ensure that we apply similar approaches to all supervisees, regardless of gender and their own anxiety. Put simply, as supervisors we would all benefit from strong supervision ourselves.

Obviously, the previously discussed evidence is not specific to supervision for EDs, and the research needs to be expanded to make sure that the same patterns apply. However, it would seem unwise to assume that anything will be different when we supervise ED clinicians. It is also important to note that we know nothing yet about the effect of an anxious supervisor. The combination of an anxious ED patient with an anxious clinician might well result in therapeutic slowing (Waller & Turner, 2016), but that slowing might be worsened still further if the supervisor is also anxious.

SUMMARY

The evidence throughout this book has indicated that exposure therapy is an effective tool in the treatment of EDs. Along with Chapter 18, this chapter has summarized the evidence that both clinicians and services need to be sure that we overcome institutional and personal factors that reduce the probability of implementing exposure therapy effectively. In this chapter, it is clear that both clinician and supervisor "drift" need to be considered and addressed. There is evidence to tell us what we omit and why. This evidence highlights the need to address our own knowledge, beliefs, attitudes, emotions, and behaviors as both clinicians and supervisors.

20

Final Summary

Exposure Therapy in the Treatment of Eating Disorders

At the beginning of this book, we stressed that EDs are a challenging set of problems to treat but that there are evidence-based psychotherapies that have the potential to help your patients recover and enjoy better quality of life. You learned that exposure therapy is a key clinical skill in reaching those goals.

Here, we summarize the key points that we have discussed in previous chapters and also identify areas for future evidence generation in the use of exposure therapy for EDs. You should remember that some of the best evidence-generating practice is likely to come from your clinical experience, so there are lessons here for all of us.

THE PRESENT STATUS OF EXPOSURE THERAPY FOR EATING DISORDERS

In the first part of this book, after a reminder about the nature of EDs (Chapter 1), you read about the different forms of exposure therapy (Chapter 2). You then read about the rationale and theory that underpin exposure therapy generally and for EDs specifically (Chapters 3 and 4) and how they can be carried over from the literature on anxiety-based disorders and uniquely applied to EDs (Chapter 5). We stressed some limitations in the literature, such as the fact that we are not entirely sure how exposure therapy works (although we are very clear that it *does* work). You will also be aware that there are not yet enough studies that have used exposure therapy for EDs in isolation.

In Part 2, we presented key clinical issues that you will need to consider when understanding the role of avoidant and safety behaviors in assessing ED patients (Chapter 6). We also used clinical examples of how to engage patients in understanding their problems and how exposure therapy could help them in changing their behaviors to overcome their ED (Chapter 7). You then read about a number of important considerations for planning and conducting exposure therapy in a range of settings (Chapters 8 and 9). Throughout, we have used case examples, so that you can see how these principles can be applied to your own patients.

In Part 3, you read about the application of exposure therapy to a range of key issues, including food, eating, weighing your patient, interpersonal and emotional issues, and body image (Chapters 10–14). We have detailed the evidence that supports each of these clinical approaches, using multiple clinical examples to show how that evidence can be put into practice to help your patients to change. Finally, we have detailed some other exposure techniques that you will likely find useful in working with specific symptom presentations (Chapter 15).

Overall, we have shown that the effective application of exposure therapy is a straightforward process if you understand the principles, prepare appropriately, and deliver the exposure appropriately—in short, if you know what this book tells you. However, we have also stressed that the place of exposure therapy for EDs is not set in stone. Indeed, there are ongoing developments in the field. We also need changes in clinical practice. Finally, there is evidence for you to generate. You will see that we have identified many areas where the evidence base for exposure in eating disorders needs to be enhanced, particularly as the field develops (e.g., the implementation of the inhibitory learning model). As you have read this book, we hope that you have been thinking about how your own clinical or research work might fill some of those gaps in the evidence base.

FUTURE DIRECTIONS IN EXPOSURE THERAPY FOR EATING DISORDERS

It is clear that we still have a long way to go in this field. The evidence base is solid in some areas but less well developed in others, with more of a reliance on the anxiety disorders literature than is desirable. Furthermore, even where there is heartening evidence that exposure therapy works for EDs, there is disheartening evidence that family, institutional factors, and clinicians can get in the way of that exposure being implemented. So what evidence should you be looking for in the future (or even adding to, through your own clinical and research work)?

Linkage to Cognitive Techniques

While we have outlined some ways in which cognitive approaches might be used to enhance exposure therapy (Chapter 16), these are largely based on clinical experience rather than empirical evidence. It remains to be determined conclusively whether cognitive methods are able to augment the benefits of exposure therapy. Further research should address this issue, using dismantling studies and considering whether there are different outcomes for different EDs. Until then, your focus should be on delivering exposure therapy to the best possible standard, using cognitive methods to enhance it only when there is a clear case to do so (and even then using the minimum cognitive element necessary to help with the effective delivery of exposure).

Ensuring That Exposure Is Used

From the evidence presented in Chapters 17 to 19, it is clear that our efforts in the future need to address factors that get in the way of exposure therapy being used. Those factors include families, institutions, teams, and individual clinicians. The common theme is that if any of these groups or individuals are intolerant of uncertainty or are risk-averse, they are likely to reduce the demands made of your patient, to the point where they make exposure therapy ineffective. This pattern is not unique to EDs, as it is well established in anxiety-based disorders. As with anxiety disorders, your goal needs to be explained to family, colleagues, and managers (as well as to the patient, of course) that exposure therapy is necessary and that its actual benefits outweigh its feared costs. Farrell, Kemp, Blakey, Meyer, and Deacon (2016) and others have stressed that we need to get clinicians to face their own fears to be effective users of exposure therapy. The future requires us all to realize the potential of exposure by ensuring that it is used effectively.

Implementation of Modern Approaches to Exposure Therapy

A key development that is underway at the time of writing this book is the adoption of more modern approaches to exposure therapy. Those approaches have been developed for anxiety-based disorders but show enormous potential to improve the speed, generalizability, and durability of exposure therapy's effects for EDs. These include the use of virtual reality approaches. However, the most important recent development has been in the implementation of approaches to exposure based on the inhibitory learning approach (e.g., Craske, Treanor, Conway, Zbozinek, & Vervliet, 2014; Reilly, Anderson, Gorrell, Schaumberg, & Anderson, 2017; Waller et al., 2019). Although the evidence for these approaches is in its infancy, we strongly recommend that you should consider adopting them, as appropriate to your patient's needs.

CONCLUSION

When you picked up this book, you probably had a broad idea of what is involved in exposure therapy for anxiety-based disorders, as well as a good foundation of knowledge in EDs. We hope that you now realize that there is a whole lot more to this therapeutic method than you assumed and that exposure therapy is a far more subtle and flexible approach than you might have realized. It is a behavioral approach that you can use on its own but is equally useful for integration into a wide range of therapies, such as CBT, dialectical behavioral therapy, specialist supportive clinical management, Maudsley Anorexia Nervosa Treatment for Adults (MANTRA), and FBT. Each of those therapies already contains elements of changing eating patterns, but they might be made more effective by turning that eating into an explicit anxiety-reduction learning experience. Exposure therapy is suitable for an equally wide range of clinicians to implement—psychologists, nurses, dietitians, occupational therapists, psychiatrists, and more. Most important, it applies to the whole range of patients with EDs, regardless of age and diagnosis.

The following are some tips that we hope will make you a better exposure therapist when working with EDs. Remember that the principles of exposure allow you to be flexible in how you apply it, so be inventive.

> **Tips for the Clinician Who Wants to Be a Better Exposure Therapist**
>
> - Use this book regularly to inform your practice. The evidence works best if we are aware of it and update ourselves regularly.
> - Always explain exposure therapy to your patients and to their families and loved ones—they are likely to understand it more than you might expect, and your explanation makes them more likely to engage with it.
> - Be responsive to your patient's needs, and shape exposure according to the symptoms and maintaining behaviors that your patient brings to therapy.
> - Adopt the inhibitory learning approach to get the best results. Remember, "mix it up" in terms of the exposure plan and make sure that exposure happens everywhere in the patient's life to have the maximum benefit.
> - Learn to tolerate your own anxiety about using exposure therapy, remembering that your patient has a better chance of recovery if you both tolerate the short-term uncertainty about delivering exposure therapy.
> - Supervision can be used to make you better at this evidence-based approach, but you will need a supervisor who is prepared to guide you clearly and to hold you to the task of delivering exposure appropriately.
> - Talk with your team about developing a culture of using exposure therapy appropriately (e.g., openly discussing weight with all patients as part of standard practice).
> - Add to the literature. When you have a new idea about how exposure therapy might work for a specific presentation, then tell others about it. This clinician-led evidence generation is particularly likely to be valuable in dealing with cases where we still have lots of evidence to generate, such as ARFID, other specified feeding or eating disorders, and purging disorder.

Finally, remember to focus on your patients' outcomes, so that you become as good a therapist as you can. Exposure therapy is a powerful method, and this book will help you to use it wisely and effectively. Come back to the book often to refresh your memory and to help you to troubleshoot to address the individual problems faced by your patients with eating disorders.

APPENDIX

Exposure Therapy: How It Can Help You With Your Eating Disorder

BACKGROUND

You have probably been given this handout by your clinician because they believe that your eating disorder would benefit from an approach called "exposure therapy." Alternatively, you might have received the handout from someone else. Maybe a relative, or someone else who has been treated for their eating disorder. If so, then you can share it with your clinician and ask if exposure is suitable for you. Either way, this handout addresses some of the questions that you might have about exposure therapy.

Exposure therapy is usually part of a broader evidence-based treatment for an eating disorder—such as cognitive-behavioral therapy (CBT) or family-based therapy (FBT). Exposure is a vital part of those therapies. In short, you are being offered a treatment that could be very helpful to you. This handout is to explain what exposure therapy involves, and how it could help you.

WHAT CAN EXPOSURE THERAPY DO FOR ME?

Exposure therapy is a key approach to helping you learn to successfully cope with the following:

- Fears about food and eating.
- Fears about weight gain.
- Interpersonal and social worries.
- Problems with emotional tolerance and avoidance of emotions.
- Negative body image.
- Recurrent binge eating episodes.
- Sensory aversions to the taste, texture, and/or smell of foods.
- Other anxiety-based disorders that you might be experiencing alongside your eating disorder.

Assuming that any or all of those experiences sound familiar to you, then please read on.

HOW DOES EXPOSURE THERAPY WORK?

Exposure therapy works by helping you learn to confront anxiety-provoking situations. If you give yourself enough time to sit with your anxiety, you will likely learn that these situations are safe and tolerable. When we are scared, we often avoid the scary thing or use "safety behaviors" to cope with our anxiety. Safety behaviors are similar to a child bringing a comforting toy or object to a situation that otherwise seems scary. Both avoidance and safety behaviors prevent you from learning two critical lessons. First, many situations that cause significant anxiety are, in fact, reasonably safe—and you can learn this if you stay in the situation. Second, you can tolerate more anxiety than you likely think. Anxiety can feel really bad, and it makes us want to avoid or use our safety behaviors to make it go away. However, your anxiety will not actually hurt you, and if you allow yourself to be anxious—you will discover that you can tolerate it better than you expect. You also may discover that your anxiety fades away. Anxiety is a bit like a school bully. The more you fear it—the more it chases you. However, when you learn to tolerate anxiety, it often fades away.

For example, you might avoid breakfast and lunch for fear of gaining weight. However, this avoidance means that you never learn what regular eating will do to your weight and you don't discover that you can handle your anxiety. In addition, you end up feeling more pressure (e.g., you end up feeling starved). And this leads you to respond in a way (e.g., binge-eating in the evening) that makes you feel even worse (e.g., you feel guilty, stuffed, and out of control). You might also gain more weight with binge eating than you would with normal eating. That puts you in a vicious cycle, because you then try to avoid food again the next day. Then, the whole pattern happens again and again and again . . .

You also might obsessively check the calories in the food you eat. This safety behavior prevents you from learning that you can eat normally even if you don't know how many calories are in your food. And because checking calories reduces your anxiety in the short term, you don't learn that you can handle your anxiety better than you think.

In summary, the avoidant or safety behaviors make you feel calmer in the short-term, but make you feel worse in the longer term. Therefore, exposure therapy means experiencing the anxiety *and* not using your avoidant or safety behaviors. In the example above, your therapist might start you off by asking you to eat breakfast. However, they would ask you to sit with the anxiety instead of using a safety behavior (like vomiting) to reduce it. That way, you can get on with the day feeling happier, with more energy, and with less chance of binge-eating later on.

A key part of this therapy is to teach you how to handle your anxiety in many different settings. That means that your therapist will be aiming to get you to experience your anxiety at different levels, in different places, and in different contexts. You learn that the world, food, your body, and all the rest are much safer than you think. So, expect to be doing work in the clinic with your therapist. But also expect to be doing exposure at home and in the wider world. You will feel the long-term benefit, once you face that short-term anxiety and feel it fading away.

WHAT IS THE EVIDENCE THAT EXPOSURE THERAPY WORKS?

In short, the evidence is very good. As long as you are prepared to tolerate your anxiety in the short term, then you will learn that feared situations are safer than expected and that you can tolerate your anxiety. In many cases, once you learn these things, anxiety fades away. To make this happen, you will have to do things that are somewhat scary. For instance, you might need to try scary foods, sit with your emotions, look at your body, etc. The more of this exposure to anxiety that you do, the more that you learn that the things you were scared of are not so scary. You will learn to deal with them far more positively (eating normally, not hiding your body, being allowed emotions, mixing with other people). You also will learn that exposure becomes easier with practice.

If you do that, then all the evidence suggests that you have an excellent chance of recovering from your eating disorder. And remember, this is not just something that happens in eating disorders. Exposure therapy is just as powerful in treating anxiety disorders. The evidence is on your side.

WHAT ELSE DO I NEED TO KNOW?

Please remember that you and the people around you might have adapted to your fear responses. For example:

- you might have covered up all the mirrors in your home.
- your parents or partner might have changed the food they buy so that you are not exposed to "scary" foods in the kitchen.
- your friends might have stopped asking you out, in case you are too scared to be somewhere with foods that feel out of control.

Everyone might be worried that you will be too distressed to cope with any changes. These things that your family and friends do to reduce your anxiety might feel helpful, but they maintain the problem in the long run. Therefore, it will be very important for you to talk with the people around you about what exposure therapy involves. Your therapist can help you with that.

One final point—you need to be an active participant in exposure therapy for your eating disorder. You will need to face your fears, with support from your therapist, family, friends, and partner. That means not avoiding or using your safety behaviors. If you take on your fears, then exposure therapy gives you the best chance of benefiting from treatment for your eating disorder.

© Becker, Farrell, & Waller (2019). Clinicians are free to copy and use this handout for clinical and teaching purposes, but please contact the authors for permission to modify or translate it.

BINGE CUE MONITORING FORM

Instructions: Please use this form to record as much information as you can whenever you notice an increased urge to binge or after you have binged.

Day & time	Where were you? What was going on around you?	What body sensations were you experiencing?	What thoughts were you having?	What emotions were you feeling?

REFERENCES

Abdallah, C. G., Averill, L. A., Akiki, T. J., Raza, M., Averill, C. L., Gomaa, H., ... Krystal, J. H. (2019). The neurobiology and pharmacotherapy of posttraumatic stress disorder. *Annual Review of Pharmacology and Toxicology, 59*, 171–189.

Abramowitz, J. S., Deacon, B. J., & Whiteside, S. P. (2011). *Exposure therapy for anxiety: Principles and practice.* New York, NY: Guilford.

Abramowitz, J. S., Taylor, S., & McKay, D. (2009). Obsessive-compulsive disorder. *The Lancet, 374*, 491–499.

Addis, M. E., & Krasnow, A. D. (2000). A national survey of practicing psychologists' attitudes towards psychotherapy treatment manuals. *Journal of Consulting and Clinical Psychology, 68*, 331–339.

Addis, M. E., & Waltz, J. (2002). Implicit and untested assumptions about the role of psychotherapy treatment manuals in evidence-based mental health practice. *Clinical Psychology: Science and Practice, 9*, 421–424.

Ahrberg, M., Trojca, D., Nasrawi, N., & Vocks, S. (2011). Body image disturbance in binge eating disorder: A review. *European Eating Disorders Review, 19*, 375–381.

American Psychiatric Association, DSM-5 Task Force. (2013). *Diagnostic and statistical manual of mental disorders* (5th ed.). Arlington, VA: American Psychiatric Publishing.

American Psychological Association. (2017). *Clinical practice guideline for the treatment of posttraumatic stress disorder (PTSD) in adults.* American Psychological Association Guideline Development Panel for the Treatment of PTSD in Adults. Retrieved from https://www.apa.org/ptsd-guideline/ptsd.pdf

Amir, N., Freshman, M., & Foa, E. B. (2000). Family distress and involvement in relatives of obsessive-compulsive disorder patients. *Journal of Anxiety Disorders, 14*, 209–217.

Anderson, L. M., Smith, K. E., Nuñez, M. C., & Farrell, N. R. (in press). Family accommodation in eating disorders: A preliminary examination of correlates with familial burden and cognitive-behavioral treatment outcome. *Eating Disorders: Journal of Treatment & Prevention.*

Arcelus, J., Mitchell, A. J., Wales, J., & Nielsen, S. (2011). Mortality rates in patients with anorexia nervosa and other eating disorders: A meta-analysis of 36 studies. *Archives of General Psychiatry, 68,* 724–731.

Barlow, D. H., & Craske, M. G. (1994). *Mastery of your anxiety and panic II.* New York, NY: Graywind.

Beat. (2015). *The costs of eating disorders: Social, health and economic impacts.* London, England: PriceWaterhouseCoopers.

Beck, A. T., Rush, A. J., Shaw, B. F., & Emery, G. (1979). *Cognitive therapy of depression.* New York, NY: Guilford.

Becker, C. B., Meyer, G., Price, J. S., Graham, M. M., Arsena, A., Armstrong, D. A., & Ramon, E. (2009). Law enforcement preferences for PTSD treatment and crisis management alternatives. *Behaviour Research and Therapy, 47,* 245–253.

Becker, C. B., & Stice, E. (2017). From efficacy to effectiveness to broad implementation: Evolution of the Body Project. *Journal of Consulting and Clinical Psychology, 85,* 767–782.

Becker, C. B., & Waller, G. (2017). The use of exposure-based strategies in treating eating disorders. In T. Wade (Ed.), *Encyclopedia of feeding and eating disorders.* Singapore: Springer.

Becker, C. B., Waller, G., & Vitousek, K. (2018, April). *Anxiety in the context of eating disorders: Petrified patients and anxious clinicians.* Invited five-hour clinical teaching day workshop presentation for the 2018 International Conference on Eating Disorders, Chicago, IL.

Becker, C. B., Zayfert, C., & Anderson, E. (2004). A survey of psychologists' attitudes towards and utilization of exposure therapy for PTSD. *Behaviour Research and Therapy, 42,* 277–292.

Benito, K. G., Machan, J., Freeman, J. B., Garcia, A. M., Walther, M., Frank, H., . . . Sapyta, J. (2018). Measuring fear change within exposures: Functionally defined habituation predicts outcome in three randomized controlled trials for pediatric OCD. *Journal of Consulting and Clinical Psychology, 86,* 615–630.

Birmingham, C., & Treasure, J. (2010). *Medical management of anorexia nervosa* (2nd ed.). Cambridge, England: Cambridge University Press.

Bongers, P., & Jansen, A. (2017). Emotional eating and Pavlovian learning: Evidence for conditioned appetitive responding to negative emotional states. *Cognition and Emotion, 31,* 284–297.

Borkovec, T. D., Alcaine, O. M., & Behar, E. (2004). Avoidance theory of worry and generalized anxiety disorder. In R. G. Heimberg, C. L. Turk, & D. S. Mennin (Eds.), *Generalized anxiety disorder: Advances in research and practice* (pp. 77–108). New York, NY: Guilford Press.

Boswell, J. F., Anderson, L. M., & Anderson, D. A. (2015). Integration of interoceptive exposure in eating disorder treatment. *Clinical Psychology: Science and Practice, 22,* 194–210.

Boswell, J. F., Farchione, T. J., Sauer-Zavala, S., Murray, H. W., Fortune, M. R., & Barlow, D. H. (2013). Anxiety sensitivity and interoceptive exposure: A transdiagnostic construct and change strategy. *Behavior Therapy, 44,* 417–431.

Botella, C., Serrano, B., Baños, R. M., & Garcia-Palacios, A. (2015). Virtual reality exposure-based therapy for the treatment of post-traumatic stress disorder: A review of its efficacy, the adequacy of the treatment protocol, and its acceptability. *Neuropsychiatric Disease and Treatment, 11*, 2533–2545.

Boutelle, K. N. (1998). The use of exposure with response prevention in a male anorexic. *Journal of Behavior Therapy and Experimental Psychiatry, 29*, 79–84.

Bowie, Jones, F. W., & Stobie, B. (2016, June). *What happens when the stabilisers come off? Exposure with and without safety-seeking behaviours in spider phobic students*. Paper presented at the British Association of Behavioural and Cognitive Psychotherapies 44th Annual Conference, Belfast, UK.

Bulik, C. M., Sullivan, P. F., Carter, F. A., McIntosh, V. V., & Joyce, P. R. (1998). The role of exposure with response prevention in the cognitive behavioral therapy for bulimia nervosa. *Psychological Medicine, 28*, 611–623.

Bun, P., Gorski, F., Grajewski, D., Wichniarek, R., & Zawadzki, P. (2017). Low-cost devices used in virtual reality exposure therapy. *Procedia Computer Science, 104*, 445–451.

Carter, F. A., McIntosh, V. V., Joyce, P. R., Sullivan, P. F., & Bulik, C. M. (2003). Role of exposure with response prevention in cognitive–behavioral therapy for bulimia nervosa: Three-year follow-up results. *International Journal of Eating Disorders, 33*, 127–135.

Cash, T .F. (1997). *The body image workbook: An 8-step program for learning to like your looks*. Oakland, CA: New Harbinger.

Channon, S., De Silva, P., Hemsley, D., & Perkins, R. (1989). A controlled trial of cognitive-behavioural and behavioural treatment of anorexia nervosa. *Behaviour Research and Therapy, 27*, 529–535.

Choy, Y., Fyer, A. J., & Lipsitz, J. D. (2007). Treatment of specific phobia in adults. *Clinical Psychology Review, 27*, 266–286.

Clark, D. M. (1999). Anxiety disorders: Why they persist and how to treat them. *Behaviour Research and Therapy, 37*, 5–27.

Clus, D., Larsen, M. E., Lemey, C., & Berrouiguet, S. (2018). The use of virtual reality in patients with eating disorders: Systematic review. *Journal of Medical Internet Research, 20*, e157.

Cooper, P. J., & Steere, J. (1995). A comparison of two psychological treatments for bulimia nervosa: Implications for models of maintenance. *Behaviour Research and Therapy, 33*, 875–885.

Cordery, H., & Waller, G. (2006). Nutritional knowledge of health care professionals working in the eating disorders. *European Eating Disorders Review, 14*, 462–467.

Cowdrey, N. D. (2014). *Perspectives on eating disorders: Attitudes to sufferers, and patient experiences of what goes on in cognitive behavioural therapy* (Doctoral dissertation). University of Sheffield, Sheffield, England.

Cowdrey, N. D., & Waller, G. (2015). Are we really delivering evidence-based treatments for eating disorders? How eating-disordered patients describe their experience of cognitive behavioural therapy. *Behaviour Research and Therapy, 75*, 72–77.

Craske, M. G., & Barlow, D. H. (2007). *Mastery of your anxiety and panic: Therapist guide* (4th ed.). New York, NY: Oxford University Press.

Craske, M. G., Kircanski, K., Zelikowsky, M., Mystkowski, J., Chowdhury, N., & Baker, A. (2008). Optimizing inhibitory learning during exposure therapy. *Behaviour Research and Therapy, 46*, 5–27.

Craske, M. G., Treanor, M., Conway, C. C., Zbozinek, T., & Vervliet, B. (2014). Maximizing exposure therapy: An inhibitory learning approach. *Behaviour Research and Therapy, 58*, 10–23.

Crisp, A. (2005). Stigmatization of and discrimination against people with eating disorders including a report of two nationwide surveys. *European Eating Disorders Review, 13*, 147–152.

Cukrowicz, K. C., Timmons, K. A., Sawyer, K., Caron, K. M., Gummelt, H. D., & Joiner, T. E., Jr. (2011). Improved treatment outcome associated with the shift to empirically supported treatments in an outpatient clinic is maintained over a ten-year period. *Professional Psychology: Research and Practice, 42*, 145–152.

Culver, N. C., Vervliet, B., & Craske, M. G. (2014). Compound extinction: Using the Rescorla–Wagner Model to maximize exposure therapy effects for anxiety disorders. *Clinical Psychological Science, 3*, 335–348.

Davison, G. C. (1968). Systematic desensitization as a counterconditioning process. *Journal of Abnormal Psychology, 73*, 91–99.

Deacon, B. J., & Farrell, N. R. (2013). Therapist barriers to the dissemination of exposure therapy. In E. A. Storch & D. McKay (Eds.), *Handbook of treating variants and complications in anxiety disorders* (pp. 363–373). New York, NY: Springer.

Deacon, B. J., Farrell, N. R., Kemp, J. J., Dixon, L. J., Sy, J. T., Zhang, A. R., & McGrath, P. B. (2013). Assessing therapist reservations about exposure therapy for anxiety disorders: The Therapist Beliefs about Exposure Scale. *Journal of Anxiety Disorders, 27*, 772–780.

Deacon, B. J., Lickel, J. J., Farrell, N. R., Kemp, J. J., & Hipol, L. J. (2013). Therapist perceptions and delivery of interoceptive exposure for panic disorder. *Journal of Anxiety Disorders, 27*, 259–264.

de la Rie, S. M., van Furth, E. F., De Koning, A., Noordenbos, G., & Donker, M. C. (2005). The quality of life of family caregivers of eating disorder patients. *Eating Disorders, 13*, 345–351.

Dennhag, I., Gibbons, M. B. C., Barber, J. P., Gallop, R., & Crits-Christoph, P. (2012). Do supervisors and independent judges agree on evaluations of therapist adherence and competence in the treatment of cocaine dependence? *Psychotherapy Research, 22*, 720–730.

Díaz-Ferrer, S., Rodríguez-Ruiz, S., Ortega-Roldán, B., Moreno-Domínguez, S., & Fernández Santaella, M. C. (2015). Testing the efficacy of pure versus guided mirror exposure in women with bulimia nervosa: A combination of neuroendocrine and psychological indices. *Journal of Behavior Therapy and Experimental Psychiatry, 48*, 1–8.

Dixon, L. J., Kemp, J. J., Farrell, N. R., Blakey, S. M., & Deacon, B. J. (2015). Interoceptive exposure exercises for social anxiety. *Journal of Anxiety Disorders, 33*, 25–34.

D'Souza Walsh, K., Davies, L., Pluckwell, H., Huffinley, H., & Waller, G. (2019). Alliance, technique, both, or more? Clinicians' views on what works in cognitive-behavioral therapy for eating disorders. *International Journal of Eating Disorders, 52*, 278–282.

Fairburn, C. G. (2008). *Cognitive behavior therapy and eating disorders.* New York, NY: Guilford.

Fairburn, C. G., & Beglin, S. J. (2008). Eating Disorder Examination Questionnaire (EDE-Q 6.0). In C. G. Fairburn (Ed.), *Cognitive behavior therapy and eating disorders* (pp. 309–314). New York, NY: Guilford.

Fairburn, C. G., Cooper, Z., Doll, H. A., O'Connor, M. E., Bohn, K., Hawker, D. M., . . . Palmer, R. L. (2009). Transdiagnostic cognitive-behavioral therapy for patients with eating disorders: A two-site trial with 60-week follow-up. *American Journal of Psychiatry, 166*, 311–319.

Fairburn, C. G., Cooper, Z., & Shafran, R. (2003). Cognitive behaviour therapy for eating disorders: A "transdiagnostic" theory and treatment. *Behaviour Research and Therapy, 41*, 509–528.

Fairburn, C. G., Cooper, Z., Shafran, R., & Wilson, G. T. (2008). Eating disorders: A transdiagnostic protocol. In D. H. Barlow (Ed.), *Clinical handbook of psychological disorders: A step-by-step treatment manual* (pp. 578–614). New York, NY: Guilford.

Fairburn, C. G., & Harrison, P. J. (2003). Eating disorders. *The Lancet, 361*, 407–416.

Fairburn, C. G., Marcus, M. D., & Wilson, G. T. (1993). Cognitive-behavioral therapy for binge eating and bulimia nervosa: A comprehensive treatment manual. In C. G. Fairburn & G. T. Wilson (Eds.), *Binge eating: Nature, assessment, and treatment* (pp. 361–404). New York, NY: Guilford.

Fairburn, C. G., Norman, P. A., Welch, S. L., O'Connor, M. E., Doll, H. A., & Peveler, R. C. (1995). A prospective study of outcome in bulimia nervosa and the long-term effects of three psychological treatments. *Archives of General Psychiatry, 52*, 304–312.

Fang, A., Sawyer, A. T., Asnaani, A., & Hofmann, S. G. (2013). Social mishap exposures for social anxiety disorder: An important treatment ingredient. *Cognitive and Behavioral Practice, 20*, 213–220.

Farrell, N. R., Bowie, O. R., Cimperman, M. C., Smith, B. E. R., Riemann, B. C., & Levinson, C. A. (2019). Exploring the preliminary effectiveness and acceptability of food-based exposure therapy for eating disorders: A case series of adult inpatients. *Journal of Experimental Psychopathology.* https://doi.org/10.1177/2043808718824886

Farrell, N. R., Brosof, L. C., Vanzhula, I. A., Christian, C., Bowie, O. R., & Levinson, C. A. (2019). Exploring mechanisms of action in exposure-based cognitive behavioral therapy for eating disorders: The role of eating-related fears and body-related safety behaviors. *Behavior Therapy.* https://doi.org/10.1016/j.beth.2019.01.008

Farrell, N. R., Deacon, B. J., Dixon, L. J., & Lickel, J. J. (2013). Theory-based training strategies for modifying practitioner concerns about exposure therapy. *Journal of Anxiety Disorders, 27*, 781–787.

Farrell, N. R., Deacon, B. J., Kemp, J. J., Dixon, L. J., & Sy, J. T. (2013). Do negative beliefs about exposure therapy cause its suboptimal delivery? An experimental investigation. *Journal of Anxiety Disorders, 27*, 763–771.

Farrell, N. R., Kemp, J. J., Blakey, S. M., Meyer, J. M., & Deacon, B. J. (2016). Targeting clinician concerns about exposure therapy: A pilot study comparing standard vs. enhanced training. *Behaviour Research and Therapy, 85*, 53–59.

Fernández, F., & Vandereycken, W. (1994). Influence of video confrontation on the self-evaluation of anorexia nervosa patients: A controlled study. *Eating Disorders, 2*, 135–140.

Festinger, L. (1962). *A theory of cognitive dissonance* (Vol. 2). Stanford, CA: Stanford University Press.

Festinger, L., & Carlsmith, J. M. (1959). Cognitive consequences of forced compliance. *Journal of Abnormal and Social Psychology, 58*, 203–210.

Foa, E. B., Hembree, E. A., & Rothbaum, B. O. (2007). *Prolonged exposure therapy for PTSD: Emotional processing of traumatic experiences therapist guide*. New York, NY: Oxford University Press.

Foa, E. B., & Kozak, M. J. (1986). Emotional processing of fear: exposure to corrective information. *Psychological Bulletin, 99*, 20–35.

Foa, E. B., & McNally, R. J. (1996). Mechanisms of change in exposure therapy. In R. Rapee (Ed.), *Current controversies in the anxiety disorders* (pp. 329–343). New York, NY: Guilford.

Foa, E. B., & Rothbaum, B. O. (1998). *Treatment manuals for practitioners: Treating the trauma of rape: Cognitive-behavioral therapy for PTSD*. New York, NY: Guilford.

Forbush, K. T., Richardson, J., & Bohrer, B. K. (2015). Clinicians' practices regarding blind versus open weighing among patients with eating disorders. *International Journal of Eating Disorders, 48*, 905–911.

Fursland, A., Erceg-Hurn, D. M., Byrne, S. M., & McEvoy, P. M. (2018). A single session assessment and psychoeducational intervention for eating disorders: Impact on treatment waitlists and eating disorder symptoms. *International Journal of Eating Disorders, 51*, 1373–1377.

García-Soriano, G., Roncero, M., Perpiñá, C., & Belloch, A. (2014). Intrusive thoughts in obsessive-compulsive disorder and eating disorder patients: A differential analysis. *European Eating Disorders Review, 22*, 191–199.

Gianini, L., Liu, Y., Wang, Y., Attia, E., Walsh, B. T., & Steinglass, J. (2015). Abnormal eating behavior in video-recorded meals in anorexia nervosa. *Eating Behaviors, 19*, 28–32.

Glasofer, D. R., Albano, A. M., Simpson, H. B., & Steinglass, J. E. (2016). Overcoming fear of eating: A case study of a novel use of exposure and response prevention. *Psychotherapy, 53*, 223–231.

Gonçalves, R., Pedrozo, A. L., Coutinho, E. S. F., Figueira, I., & Ventura, P. (2012). Efficacy of virtual reality exposure therapy in the treatment of PTSD: A systematic review. *PLOS ONE, 7*(12), e48469.

Graves, T. A., Tabri, N., Thompson-Brenner, H., Franko, D. L., Eddy, K. T., Bourion-Bedes, S., . . . Thomas, J. J. (2017). A meta-analysis of the relation between therapeutic alliance and treatment outcome in eating disorders. *International Journal of Eating Disorders, 50*, 323–340.

Griffen, T. C., Naumann, E., & Hildebrandt, T. (2018). Mirror exposure therapy for body image disturbances and eating disorders: A review. *Clinical Psychology Review, 65*, 163–174.

Grilo, C. M., Crosby, R. D., Masheb, R. M., White, M. A., Peterson, C. B., Wonderlich, S. A., . . . Mitchell, J. E. (2009). Overvaluation of shape and weight in binge eating disorder, bulimia nervosa, and sub-threshold bulimia nervosa. *Behaviour Research and Therapy, 47*, 692–696.

Grove, W. M., Zald, D. H., Lebow, B. S., Snitz, B. E., & Nelson, C. (2000). Clinical versus mechanical prediction: A meta-analysis. *Psychological Assessment, 12*, 19–30.

Gutiérrez-Maldonado, J., Ferrer-García, M., Caqueo-Urízar, A., & Moreno, E. (2010). Body image in eating disorders: The influence of exposure to virtual-reality environments. *Cyberpsychology, Behavior, and Social Networking, 13*, 521–531.

Harned, M. S., Dimeff, L. A., Woodcock, E. A., & Contreras, I. (2013). Predicting adoption of exposure therapy in a randomized controlled dissemination trial. *Journal of Anxiety Disorders, 27*, 754–762.

Harned, M. S., Korslund, K. E., Foa, E. B., & Linehan, M. M. (2012). Treating PTSD in suicidal and self-injuring women with borderline personality disorder: Development and preliminary evaluation of a dialectical behavior therapy prolonged exposure protocol. *Behaviour Research and Therapy, 50*, 381–386.

Heatherton, T. F., & Baumeister, R. F. (1991). Binge eating as escape from self-awareness. *Psychological Bulletin, 110*, 86–108.

Herbert, B. M., Muth, E. R., Pollatos, O., & Herbert, C. (2012). Interoception across modalities: On the relationship between cardiac awareness and the sensitivity for gastric functions. *PLOS ONE, 7*(5), e36646.

Highet, N., Thompson, M., & King, R. M. (2005). The experience of living with a person with an eating disorder: The impact on the carers. *Eating Disorders, 13*, 327–344.

Hilbert, A., & Tuschen-Caffier, B. (2004). Body image interventions in cognitive-behavioural therapy of binge-eating disorder: A component analysis. *Behaviour Research and Therapy, 42*, 1325–1339.

Hilbert, A., Tuschen-Caffier, B., & Vögele, C. (2002). Effects of prolonged and repeated body image exposure in binge-eating disorder. *Journal of Psychosomatic Research, 52*, 137–144.

Hildebrandt, T., Bacow, T., Markella, M., & Loeb, K. L. (2012). Anxiety in anorexia nervosa and its management using family-based treatment. *European Eating Disorders Review, 20*, e1–e16.

Hildebrandt, T., Loeb, K., Troupe, S., & Delinsky, S. (2012). Adjunctive mirror exposure for eating disorders: A randomized controlled pilot study. *Behaviour Research and Therapy, 50*, 797–804.

Hipol, L. J., & Deacon, B. J. (2013). Dissemination of evidence-based practices for anxiety disorders in Wyoming: A survey of practicing psychotherapists. *Behavior Modification, 37*, 170–188.

Hofmann, S. G. (2008). Cognitive processes during fear acquisition and extinction in animals and humans: Implications for exposure therapy of anxiety disorders. *Clinical Psychology Review, 28*, 199–210.

Hoyer, J., & Beesdo-Baum, K. (2012). Prolonged imaginal exposure based on worry scenarios. In P. Neudeck & H.-U. Wittchen (Eds.), *Exposure therapy* (pp. 245–260). New York, NY: Springer.

Institute of Medicine. (2001). *Crossing the quality chasm: A new health system for the 21st century*. Washington, DC: National Academy Press.

Jacoby, R. J., & Abramowitz, J. S. (2016). Inhibitory learning approaches to exposure therapy: A critical review and translation to obsessive-compulsive disorder. *Clinical Psychology Review, 49*, 28–40.

Jansen, A. (1998). A learning model of binge eating: Cue reactivity and cue exposure. *Behaviour Research and Therapy, 36*, 257–272.

Jansen, A., Bollen, D., Tuschen-Caffier, B., Roefs, A., Tanghe, A., & Braet, C. (2008). Mirror exposure reduces body dissatisfaction and anxiety in obese adolescents: A pilot study. *Appetite, 51*, 214–217.

Jansen, A., Broekmate, J., & Heymans, M. (1992). Cue-exposure vs self-control in the treatment of binge eating: A pilot study. *Behaviour Research and Therapy, 30*, 235–241.

Jansen, A., Schyns, G., Bongers, P., & van den Akker, K. (2016). From lab to clinic: Extinction of cued cravings to reduce overeating. *Physiology & Behavior, 162*, 174–180.

Jansen, A., & Van den Hout, M. (1991). On being led into temptation: "Counterregulation" of dieters after smelling a "preload." *Addictive Behaviors, 16*, 247–253.

Jansen, A., Van den Hout, M. A., De Loof, C., Zandbergen, J., & Griez, E. (1989). A case of bulimia successfully treated by cue exposure. *Journal of Behavior Therapy and Experimental Psychiatry, 20*, 327–332.

Jansen, A., Voorwinde, V., Hoebink, Y., Rekkers, M., Martijn, C., & Mulkens, S. (2016). Mirror exposure to increase body satisfaction: Should we guide the focus of attention towards positively or negatively evaluated body parts? *Journal of Behavior Therapy and Experimental Psychiatry, 50*, 90–96.

Kaye, W. H., Bulik, C. M., Thornton, L., Barbarich, N., & Masters, K. (2004). Comorbidity of anxiety disorders with anorexia and bulimia nervosa. *American Journal of Psychiatry, 161*, 2215–2221.

Keel, P. K., Dorer, D. J., Franko, D. L., Jackson, S. C., & Herzog, D. B. (2005). Postremission predictors of relapse in women with eating disorders. *American Journal of Psychiatry, 162*, 2263–2268.

Kendall, P. C., Comer, J. S., Marker, C. D., Creed, T. A., Puliafico, A. C., Hughes, A. A., ... Hudson, J. (2009). In-session exposure tasks and therapeutic alliance across the treatment of childhood anxiety disorders. *Journal of Consulting and Clinical Psychology, 77*, 517–525

Kennedy, S. H., Katz, R., Neitzert, C. S., Ralevski, E., & Mendlowitz, S. (1995). Exposure with response prevention treatment of anorexia nervosa-bulimic subtype and bulimia nervosa. *Behaviour Research and Therapy, 33*, 685–689.

Keum, B., Jeen, Y. T., Park, S. C., Seo, Y. S., Kim, Y. S., Chun, H. J., ... Ryu, H. S. (2010). Proctocolitis caused by coffee enemas. *American Journal of Gastroenterology, 105*, 229–230.

Key, A., George, C. L., Beattie, D., Stammers, K., Lacey, H., & Waller, G. (2002). Body image treatment within an inpatient program for anorexia nervosa: The role of mirror exposure in the desensitization process. *International Journal of Eating Disorders, 31*, 185–190.

Knowles, K. A., & Olatunji, B. O. (2019). Enhancing inhibitory learning: The utility of variability in exposure. *Cognitive and Behavioral Practice, 26*, 186–200.

Leitenberg, H., Rosen, J. C., Gross, J., Nudelman, S., & Vara, L. S. (1988). Exposure plus response-prevention treatment of bulimia nervosa. *Journal of Consulting and Clinical Psychology, 56*, 535–541.

Levinson, C. A., & Byrne, M. (2015). The Fear of Food Measure: A novel measure for use in exposure therapy for eating disorders. *International Journal of Eating Disorders, 48*, 271–283.

Levinson, C. A., Rapp, J., & Riley, E. N. (2014). Addressing the fear of fat: Extending imaginal exposure therapy for anxiety disorders to anorexia nervosa. *Eating and Weight Disorders—Studies on Anorexia, Bulimia and Obesity, 19*, 521–524.

Levinson, C. A., Rodebaugh, T. L., Fewell, L., Kass, A. E., Riley, E. N., Stark, L., ... Lenze, E. J. (2015). D-cycloserine facilitation of exposure therapy improves weight regain in patients with anorexia nervosa: A pilot randomized controlled trial. *Journal of Clinical Psychiatry, 76*, 787–793.

Levinson, C. A., Sala, M., Fewell, L., Brosof, L. C., Fournier, L., & Lenze, E. J. (2018). Meal and snack-time eating disorder cognitions predict eating disorder behaviors and vice versa in a treatment seeking sample: A mobile technology based ecological momentary assessment study. *Behaviour Research and Therapy, 105*, 36–42.

Levinson, C. A., Vanzhula, I., Brosof, L., Michelson, L., Calebs, B., Christian, C., & Fewell, L. (2017, November). *A trial of online imaginal exposure therapy for eating disorder related fears in individuals with anorexia nervosa*. Paper presented at the meeting of Association for Behavioral and Cognitive Therapies, San Diego, CA.

Levinson, C. A., Zerwas, S., Calebs, B., Forbush, K., Kordy, H., Watson, H., . . . Runfola, C. D. (2017). The core symptoms of bulimia nervosa, anxiety, and depression: A network analysis. *Journal of Abnormal Psychology, 126*, 340–354.

Levita, L., Salas Duhne, P. G., Girling, C., & Waller, G. (2016). Facets of clinicians' anxiety and the delivery of cognitive-behaviour therapy. *Behaviour Research and Therapy, 77*, 157–161.

Lewer, M., Kosfelder, J., Michalak, J., Schroeder, D., Nasrawi, N., & Vocks, S. (2017). Effects of a cognitive-behavioral exposure-based body image therapy for overweight females with binge eating disorder: A pilot study. *Journal of Eating Disorders, 5*, e43.

Linehan, M. M. (1993). *Cognitive-behavioral treatment of borderline personality disorder*. New York, NY: Guilford.

Lock, J., & Le Grange, D. (2013). *Treatment manual for anorexia nervosa: A family-based approach*. New York, NY: Guilford.

Luethcke, C. A., McDaniel, L., & Becker, C. B. (2011). A comparison of mindfulness, nonjudgmental, and cognitive dissonance-based approaches to mirror exposure. *Body Image, 8*, 251–258.

Luo, X., Nuttall, A. K., Locke, K. D., & Hopwood, C. J. (2018). Dynamic longitudinal relations between binge eating symptoms and severity and style of interpersonal problems. *Journal of Abnormal Psychology, 127*, 30–42.

Martinez-Mallén, E., Castro-Fornieles, J., Lázaro, L., Moreno, E., Morer, A., Font, E., . . . Toro, J. (2007). Cue exposure in the treatment of resistant adolescent bulimia nervosa. *International Journal of Eating Disorders, 40*, 596–601.

Marzola, E., Nasser, J. A., Hashim, S. A., Shih, P. B., & Kaye, W. H. (2013). Nutritional rehabilitation in anorexia nervosa: Review of the literature and implications for treatment. *BMC Psychiatry, 13*, 290–103.

Mavissakalian, M. (1982). Anorexia nervosa treated with response prevention and prolonged exposure. *Behaviour Research and Therapy, 20*, 27–31.

McHugh, R. K., Smits, J. A., & Otto, M. W. (2009). Empirically supported treatments for panic disorder. *Psychiatric Clinics of North America, 32*, 593–610.

McIntosh, V. V. W., Carter, F. A., Bulik, C. M., Frampton, C. M. A., & Joyce, P. R. (2011). Five-year outcome of cognitive behavioral therapy and exposure with response prevention for bulimia nervosa. *Psychological Medicine, 41*, 1061–1071.

McManus, F., Waller, G., & Chadwick, P. (1996). Biases in the processing of different forms of threat in bulimic and comparison women. *Journal of Nervous and Mental Disease, 184*, 547–554.

McMillan, D., & Lee, R. (2010). A systematic review of behavioral experiments vs. exposure alone in the treatment of anxiety disorders: A case of exposure while wearing the emperor's new clothes? *Clinical Psychology Review, 30*, 467–478.

Meehl, P. E. (1954). *Clinical versus statistical prediction: A theoretical analysis and a review of the evidence.* Minneapolis, MN: University of Minnesota Press.

Meehl, P. E. (1973). Why I do not attend case conferences. In P. E. Meehl, *Psychodiagnosis: Selected papers* (pp. 225–302). Minneapolis, MN: University of Minnesota Press.

Meehl, P. E. (1986). Causes and effects of my disturbing little book. *Journal of Personality Assessment, 50*, 370–375.

Merlo, L. J., Lehmkuhl, H. D., Geffken, G. R., & Storch, E. A. (2009). Decreased family accommodation associated with improved therapy outcome in pediatric obsessive-compulsive disorder. *Journal of Consulting and Clinical Psychology, 77*, 355–360.

Merwin, R. M., Zucker, N. L., Lacy, J. L., & Elliott, C. A. (2010). Interoceptive awareness in eating disorders: Distinguishing lack of clarity from non-acceptance of internal experience. *Cognition and Emotion, 24*, 892–902.

Meyer, J. M., Farrell, N. R., Kemp, J. J., Blakey, S. M., & Deacon, B. J. (2014). Why do clinicians exclude anxious clients from exposure therapy? *Behaviour Research and Therapy, 54*, 49–53.

Meyerbröker, K., & Emmelkamp, P. M. (2010). Virtual reality exposure therapy in anxiety disorders: A systematic review of process-and-outcome studies. *Depression and Anxiety, 27*, 933–944.

Mineka, S., & Thomas, C. (1999). Mechanisms of change in exposure therapy for anxiety disorders. In T. Dalgleish & M. J. Power (Eds.), *Handbook of cognition and emotion* (pp. 747–764). New York, NY: Wiley.

Moreno-Domínguez, S., Rodríguez-Ruiz, S., Fernández-Santaella, M. C., Jansen, A., & Tuschen-Caffier, B. (2012). Pure versus guided mirror exposure to reduce body dissatisfaction: A preliminary study with university women. *Body Image, 9*, 285–288.

Morgan, J. F., Lazarova, S., Schelhase, M., & Saeidi, S. (2014). Ten session body image therapy: Efficacy of a manualised body image therapy. *European Eating Disorders Review, 22*, 66–71.

Mulkens, S., de Vos, C., de Graaff, A., & Waller, G. (2018). To deliver or not to deliver cognitive behavioral therapy for eating disorders: Replication and extension of our understanding of why therapists fail to do what they should do. *Behaviour Research and Therapy, 106*, 57–63.

Murray, S. B., Strober, M., Craske, M. G., Griffiths, S., Levinson, C. A., & Strigo, I. A. (2018). Fear as a translational mechanism in the psychopathology of anorexia nervosa. *Neuroscience & Biobehavioral Reviews, 95*, 383–395.

Murray, S. B., Treanor, M., Liao, B., Loeb, K. L., Griffiths, S., & Le Grange, D. (2016). Extinction theory & anorexia nervosa: Deepening therapeutic mechanisms. *Behaviour Research and Therapy, 87*, 1–10.

National Institute for Health and Care Excellence. (2017). *Eating disorders: Recognition and treatment.* London, UK: Author.

Nelson, E. A., Deacon, B. J., Lickel, J. J., & Sy, J. T. (2010). Targeting the probability versus cost of feared outcomes in public speaking anxiety. *Behaviour Research and Therapy, 48*, 282–289.

Neumark-Sztainer, D., Paxton, S. J., Hannan, P. J., Haines, J., & Story, M. (2006). Does body satisfaction matter? Five-year longitudinal associations between body satisfaction and health behaviors in adolescent females and males. *Journal of Adolescent Health, 39*, 244–251.

Nicely, T. A., Lane-Loney, S., Masciulli, E., Hollenbeak, C. S., & Ornstein, R. M. (2014). Prevalence and characteristics of avoidant/restrictive food intake disorder in a cohort of young patients in day treatment for eating disorders. *Journal of Eating Disorders*, *2*, e21.

Nicholls, D., Christie, D., Randall, L., & Lask, B. (2001). Selective eating: Symptom, disorder or normal variant? *Clinical and Child Psychology and Psychiatry*, *6*, 257–270.

Norris, D. L. (1984). The effects of mirror confrontation on self estimation of body dimensions in anorexia nervosa, bulimia and two control groups. *Psychological Medicine*, *14*, 835–842.

Olatunji, B. O., Cisler, J. M., & Deacon, B. J. (2010). Efficacy of cognitive behavioral therapy for anxiety disorders: A review of meta-analytic findings. *Psychiatric Clinics of North America*, *33*, 557–577.

Olatunji, B. O., Deacon, B. J., & Abramowitz, J. S. (2009). The cruelest cure? Ethical issues in the implementation of exposure-based treatments. *Cognitive and Behavioral Practice*, *16*, 172–180.

Öst, L. G., Havnen, A., Hansen, B., & Kvale, G. (2015). Cognitive behavioral treatments of obsessive–compulsive disorder. A systematic review and meta-analysis of studies published 1993–2014. *Clinical Psychology Review*, *40*, 156–169.

Padesky, C. A., & Mooney, K. A. (1990). Presenting the cognitive model to clients. *International Cognitive Therapy Newsletter*, *6*, 13–14. Retrieved from www.padesky.com

Parker, Z. J., & Waller, G. (2017). Development and validation of the Negative Attitudes Towards CBT Scale. *Behavioural and Cognitive Psychotherapy*, *45*, 629–646.

Parsons, T. D., & Rizzo, A. A. (2008). Affective outcomes of virtual reality exposure therapy for anxiety and specific phobias: A meta-analysis. *Journal of Behavior Therapy and Experimental Psychiatry*, *39*, 250–261.

Perkins, S., Winn, S., Murray, J., Murphy, R., & Schmidt, U. (2004). A qualitative study of the experience of caring for a person with bulimia nervosa: Part 1. The emotional impact of caring. *International Journal of Eating Disorders*, *36*, 256–268.

Pittig, A., Kotter, R., & Hoyer, J. (2019). The struggle of behavioral therapists with exposure: Self-reported practicability, negative beliefs, and therapist distress about exposure-based interventions. *Behavior Therapy*, *50*, 353–366.

Ponniah, K., & Hollon, S. D. (2008). Empirically supported psychological interventions for social phobia in adults: A qualitative review of randomized controlled trials. *Psychological Medicine*, *38*, 3–14.

Rachman, S. J. (1977). The conditioning theory of fear acquisition: A critical examination. *Behaviour Research and Therapy*, *15*, 375–387.

Rachman, S., Radomsky, A. S., & Shafran, R. (2008). Safety behaviour: A reconsideration. *Behaviour Research and Therapy*, *46*, 163–173.

Rauch, S., & Foa, E. (2006). Emotional Processing Theory (EPT) and exposure therapy for PTSD. *Journal of Contemporary Psychotherapy*, *36*, 61–65.

Reas, D. L., Whisenhunt, B. L., Netemeyer, R., & Williamson, D. A. (2002). Development of the Body Checking Questionnaire: A self-report measure of body checking behaviors. *International Journal of Eating Disorders*, *31*, 324–333.

Reilly, E. R., Anderson, L. M., Gorrell, S., Schaumberg, K., & Anderson, D. A. (2017). Expanding exposure-based interventions for eating disorders. *International Journal of Eating Disorders*, *50*, 1137–1141.

Reiss, S. (1991). Expectancy model of fear, anxiety, and panic. *Clinical Psychology Review, 11*, 141–153.

Resick, P. A., Nishith, P., Weaver, T. L., Astin, M. C., & Feuer, C. A. (2002). A comparison of cognitive-processing therapy with prolonged exposure and a waiting condition for the treatment of chronic posttraumatic stress disorder in female rape victims. *Journal of Consulting and Clinical Psychology, 70*, 867–879.

Rienecke, R. D., Lebow, J., Lock, J., & Le Grange, D. (2017). Family profiles of expressed emotion in adolescent patients with anorexia nervosa and their parents. *Journal of Clinical Child & Adolescent Psychology, 46*, 428–436.

Robinson, P., Hellier, J., Barrett, B., Barzdaitiene, D., Bateman, A., Bogaardt, A., ... Kern, N. (2016). The NOURISHED randomised controlled trial comparing mentalisation-based treatment for eating disorders (MBT-ED) with specialist supportive clinical management (SSCM-ED) for patients with eating disorders and symptoms of borderline personality disorder. *Trials, 17*, 549.

Rohde, P., Stice, E., & Marti, C. N. (2015). Development and predictive effects of eating disorder risk factors during adolescence: Implications for prevention efforts. *International Journal of Eating Disorders, 48*, 187–198.

Rosen, J. C., & Leitenberg, H. (1982). Bulimia nervosa: Treatment with exposure and response prevention. *Behavior Therapy, 13*, 117–124.

Rosen, J. C., Srebnik, D., Saltzberg, E., & Wendt, S. (1991). Development of a body image avoidance questionnaire. *Psychological Assessment: A Journal of Consulting and Clinical Psychology, 3*, 32–37.

Rushford, N., & Ostermeyer, A. (1997). Body image disturbances and their change with videofeedback in anorexia nervosa. *Behaviour Research and Therapy, 35*, 389–398.

Salkovskis, P. M. (1991). the importance of behavior in the maintenance of anxiety and panic: A cognitive account. *Behavioural Psychotherapy, 19*, 6–19.

Salkovskis, P. M., Wroe, A. L., Gledhill, A., Morrison, N., Forrester, E., Richards, C., ... Thorpe, S. (2000). Responsibility attitudes and interpretations are characteristic of obsessive compulsive disorder. *Behaviour Research and Therapy, 38*, 347–372.

Schmidt, U., & Treasure, J. (2006). Anorexia nervosa: Valued and visible. A cognitive-interpersonal maintenance model and its implications for research and practice. *British Journal of Clinical Psychology, 45*, 343–366.

Schumacher, S., Gaudlitz, K., Plag, J., Miller, R., Kirschbaum, C., Fehm, L., ... Ströhle, A. (2014). Who is stressed? A pilot study of salivary cortisol and alpha amylase concentrations in agoraphobic patients and their novice therapists undergoing in vivo exposure. *Psychoneuroendocrinology, 49*, 280–289.

Schumacher, S., Miller, R., Fehm, L., Kirschbaum, C., Fydrich, T., & Ströhle, A. (2015). Therapists' and patients' stress responses during graduated versus flooding in vivo exposure in the treatment of specific phobia: A preliminary observational study. *Psychiatry Research, 230*, 668–675.

Schyns, G., van den Akker, K., Roefs, A., Hilberath, R., & Jansen, A. (2018). What works better? Food cue exposure aiming at the habituation of eating desires or food cue exposure aiming at the violation of overeating expectancies? *Behaviour Research and Therapy, 102*, 1–7.

Sepulveda, A. R., Kyriacou, O., & Treasure, J. (2009). Development and validation of the Accommodation and Enabling Scale for Eating Disorders (AESED) for caregivers in eating disorders. *BMC Health Services Research, 9*, 171.

Shafran, R., & Robinson, P. (2004). Thought-shape fusion in eating disorders. *British Journal of Clinical Psychology*, *43*, 399–408.

Simpson, H. B., Wetterneck, C. T., Cahill, S. P., Steinglass, J. E., Franklin, M. E., Leonard, R. C., . . . Riemann, B. C. (2013). Treatment of obsessive-compulsive disorder complicated by comorbid eating disorders. *Cognitive Behaviour Therapy*, *42*, 64–76.

Simpson-Southward, C., Waller, G., & Hardy, G. (2016). Supervision for treatment of depression: An experimental study of the role of therapist gender and anxiety. *Behaviour Research and Therapy*, *77*, 17–22.

Simpson Southward, C., Waller, G., & Hardy, G. (2017). How do we know what makes for "best practice" in clinical supervision for psychological therapists? A content analysis of supervisory models and approaches. *Clinical Psychology and Psychotherapy*, *24*, 1228–1245.

Slater, L. (2003, November 2). The cruelest cure. *The New York Times Magazine*, p. 34. Retrieved from https://www.nytimes.com/2003/11/02/magazine/the-cruelest-cure.html

Smith, K. E., Mason, T. B., Crosby, R. D., Cao, L., Leonard, R. C., Wetterneck, C. T., . . . Moessner, M. (2018). A comparative network analysis of eating disorder psychopathology and co-occurring depression and anxiety symptoms before and after treatment. *Psychological Medicine*, *15*, 1–11.

Sripada, R. K., & Rauch, S. A. (2015). Between-session and within-session habituation in Prolonged Exposure Therapy for posttraumatic stress disorder: A hierarchical linear modeling approach. *Journal of Anxiety Disorders*, *30*, 81–87.

Stanley, M. A., & Averill, P. M. (1998). Psychosocial treatments for obsessive-compulsive disorder: Clinical applications. In R. P. Swinson (Ed.), *Obsessive–compulsive disorder: Theory, research and treatment* (pp. 277–297). New York, NY: Guilford.

Steinglass, J., Albano, A. M., Simpson, H. B., Carpenter, K., Schebendach, J., & Attia, E. (2012). Fear of food as a treatment target: Exposure and response prevention for anorexia nervosa in an open series. *International Journal of Eating Disorders*, *45*, 615–621.

Steinglass, J. E., Albano, A. M., Simpson, H. B., Wang, Y., Zou, J., Attia, E., & Walsh, B. T. (2014). Confronting fear using exposure and response prevention for anorexia nervosa: A randomized controlled pilot study. *International Journal of Eating Disorders*, *47*, 174–180.

Steinglass, J., Sysko, R., Schebendach, J., Broft, A., Strober, M., & Walsh, B. T. (2007). The application of exposure therapy and D-cycloserine to the treatment of anorexia nervosa: A preliminary trial. *Journal of Psychiatric Practice*, *13*, 238–245.

Steketee, G., Frost, R., & Bogart, K. (1996). The Yale-Brown Obsessive Compulsive Scale: Interview versus self-report. *Behaviour Research and Therapy*, *34*, 675–684.

Stice, E., Rohde, P., Butryn, M., Menke, K. S., & Marti, C. N. (2015). Randomized controlled pilot trial of a novel dissonance-based group treatment for eating disorders. *Behaviour Research and Therapy*, *65*, 67–75.

Steiger, H., Gauvin, L., Jabalpurwala, S., Séguin, J. R., & Stotland, S. (1999). Hypersensitivity to social interactions in bulimic syndromes: Relationship to binge eating. *Journal of Consulting and Clinical Psychology*, *67*, 765–775.

Stobie, B., Taylor, T., Quigley, A., Ewing, S., & Salkovskis, P. M. (2007). "Contents may vary": A pilot study of treatment histories of OCD patients. *Behavioural and Cognitive Psychotherapy*, *35*, 273–282.

Storch, E. A., Merlo, L. J., Larson, M. J., Marien, W. E., Geffken, G. R., Jacob, M. L., . . . Murphy, T. K. (2008). Clinical features associated with treatment-resistant pediatric obsessive-compulsive disorder. *Comprehensive Psychiatry, 49*, 35–42.

Swinbourne, J. M., & Touyz, S. W. (2007). The co-morbidity of eating disorders and anxiety disorders: A review. *European Eating Disorders Review, 15*, 253–274.

Szmukler, G. I., Eisler, I., Russell, G. F. M., & Dare, C. (1985). Anorexia nervosa, parental "expressed emotion" and dropping out of treatment. *The British Journal of Psychiatry, 147*, 265–271.

Thompson-Hollands, J., Edson, A., Tompson, M. C., & Comer, J. S. (2014). Family involvement in the psychological treatment of obsessive–compulsive disorder: A meta-analysis. *Journal of Family Psychology, 28*, 287–298.

Tobin, D. L., Banker, J. D., Weisberg, L., & Bowers, W. (2007). I know what you did last summer (and it was not CBT): A factor analytic model of international psychotherapeutic practice in the eating disorders. *International Journal of Eating Disorders, 40*, 754–757.

Toli, A., Webb, T. L., & Hardy, G. E. (2016). Does forming implementation intentions help people with mental health problems to achieve goals? A meta-analysis of experimental studies with clinical and analogue samples. *British Journal of Clinical Psychology, 55*, 69–90.

Toro, J., Cervera, M., Feliu, M. H., Garriga, N., Jou, M., Martinez, E., & Toro, E. (2003). Cue exposure in the treatment of resistant bulimia nervosa. *International Journal of Eating Disorders, 34*, 227–234.

Treasure, J., Gavan, K., Todd, G., & Schmidt, U. (2003). Changing the environment in eating disorders: Working with carers/families to improve motivation and facilitate change. *European Eating Disorders Review, 11*, 25–37.

Trentowska, M., Svaldi, J., Blechert, J., & Tuschen-Caffier, B. (2017). Does habituation really happen? Investigation of psycho-biological responses to body exposure in bulimia nervosa. *Behaviour Research and Therapy, 90*, 111–122.

Trentowska, M., Svaldi, J., & Tuschen-Caffier, B. (2014). Efficacy of body exposure as treatment component for patients with eating disorders. *Journal of Behavior Therapy and Experimental Psychiatry, 45*, 178–185.

Trottier, K., Carter, J. C., MacDonald, D. E., McFarlane, T., & Olmsted, M. P. (2015). Adjunctive graded body image exposure for eating disorders: A randomized controlled initial trial in clinical practice. *International Journal of Eating Disorders, 48*, 494–504.

Trottier, K., MacDonald, D. E., McFarlane, T., Carter, J., & Olmsted, M. P. (2015). Body checking, body avoidance, and the core cognitive psychopathology of eating disorders: Is there a unique relationship? *Advances in Eating Disorders: Theory, Research, and Practice, 3*, 288–299.

Tucker, T. (2006). *The great starvation experiment: The heroic men who starved so that millions could live*. New York, NY: Simon & Schuster.

Turner, H., Marshall, E., Stopa, L., & Waller, G. (2015). Cognitive-behavioural therapy for outpatients with eating disorders: Effectiveness for a transdiagnostic group in a routine clinical setting. *Behaviour Research and Therapy, 68*, 70–75.

Turner, H., Tatham, M., Lant, M., Mountford, V. A., & Waller, G. (2014). Clinicians' concerns about delivering cognitive-behavioural therapy for eating disorders. *Behaviour Research and Therapy, 57*, 38–42.

Vall, E., & Wade, T. D. (2015). Predictors of treatment outcome in individuals with eating disorders: A systematic review and meta-analysis. *International Journal of Eating Disorders, 48*, 946–971.

Van den Berg, P., Neumark-Sztainer, D., Hannan, P. J., & Haines, J. (2007). Is dieting advice from magazines helpful or harmful? Five-year associations with weight-control behaviors and psychological outcomes in adolescents. *Pediatrics, 119*, e30–e37.

van Minnen, A., Hendricks, L., & Olff, M. (2010). When do trauma experts choose exposure therapy for PTSD patients? A controlled study of therapist and patient factors. *Behaviour Research and Therapy, 48*, 312–320.

Vervliet, B., Craske, M. G., & Hermans, D. (2013). Fear extinction and relapse: State of the art. *Annual Review of Clinical Psychology, 9*, 215–248.

Vitousek, K. B. (2019). *Pros and cons of transdiagnostic thinking: Examples from the eating disorder field.* World Congress of Behavioural and Cognitive Psychotherapy, Berlin, July.

Vocks, S., Kosfelder, J., Wucherer, M., & Wächter, A. (2008). Does habitual body avoidance and checking behavior influence the decrease of negative emotions during body exposure in eating disorders? *Psychotherapy Research, 18*, 412–419.

Vocks, S., Legenbauer, T., Wächter, A., Wucherer, M., & Kosfelder, J. (2007). What happens in the course of body exposure? Emotional, cognitive, and physiological reactions to mirror confrontation in eating disorders. *Journal of Psychosomatic Research, 62*, 231–239.

Vocks, S., Schulte, D., Busch, M., Grönemeyer, D., Herpertz, S., & Suchan, B. (2011). Changes in neuronal correlates of body image processing by means of cognitive-behavioural body image therapy for eating disorders: A randomized controlled fMRI study. *Psychological Medicine, 41*, 1651–1663.

Vocks, S., Wächter, A., Wucherer, M., & Kosfelder, J. (2008). Look at yourself: Can body image therapy affect the cognitive and emotional response to seeing oneself in the mirror in eating disorders? *European Eating Disorders Review, 16*, 147–154.

Wade, T. D., Bergin, J. L., Martin, N. G., Gillespie, N. A., & Fairburn, C. G. (2006). A transdiagnostic approach to understanding eating disorders. *Journal of Nervous and Mental Disease, 194*, 510–517.

Wald, J., & Taylor, S. (2007). Efficacy of interoceptive exposure therapy combined with trauma-related exposure therapy for posttraumatic stress disorder: A pilot study. *Journal of Anxiety Disorders, 21*, 1050–1060.

Wald, J., & Taylor, S. (2008). Responses to interoceptive exposure in people with posttraumatic stress disorder (PTSD): A preliminary analysis of induced anxiety reactions and trauma memories and their relationship to anxiety sensitivity and PTSD symptom severity. *Cognitive Behaviour Therapy, 37*, 90–100.

Walfish, S., McAlister, B., O'Donnel, P., & Lambert, M. (2012). An investigation of self-assessment bias in mental health providers. *Psychological Reports, 110*, 1–6.

Waller, G. (2008). A "trans-transdiagnostic" model of the eating disorders: A new way to open the egg? *European Eating Disorders Review, 16*, 165–172.

Waller, G. (2009). Evidence-based treatment and therapist drift. *Behaviour Research and Therapy, 47*, 119–127.

Waller, G., Cordery, H., Corstorphine, E., Hinrichsen, H., Lawson, R., Mountford, V., & Russell, K. (2007). *Cognitive-behavioral therapy for eating disorders: A comprehensive treatment guide.* Cambridge, England: Cambridge University Press.

Waller, G., Evans, J., & Pugh, M. (2013). Food for thought: A pilot study of the pros and cons of changing eating patterns within cognitive-behavioural therapy for the eating disorders. *Behaviour Research and Therapy, 51,* 519–525.

Waller, G., & Mountford, V. A. (2015). Weighing patients within cognitive-behavioural therapy for eating disorders: How, when and why. *Behaviour Research and Therapy, 70,* 1–10.

Waller, G., Mountford, V. A., Tatham, M., Turner, H., Gabriel, C., & Webber, R. (2013). Attitudes towards psychotherapy manuals among clinicians treating eating disorders. *Behaviour Research and Therapy, 51,* 840–844.

Waller, G., & Raykos, B. (2019). Behavioral interventions in the treatment of eating disorders. *Psychiatric Clinics of North America, 42,* 181–191.

Waller, G., Stringer, H, & Meyer, C. (2012). What cognitive-behavioral techniques do therapists report using when delivering cognitive-behavioral therapy for the eating disorders? *Journal of Consulting and Clinical Psychology, 80,* 171–175.

Waller, G., Tatham, M., Turner, H., Mountford, V. A., Bennetts, A., Bramwell, K., . . . Ingram, L. (2018). A 10-session cognitive-behavioral therapy (CBT-T) for eating disorders: Outcomes from a case series of non-underweight adult patients. *International Journal of Eating Disorders, 51,* 262–269.

Waller, G., & Turner, H. (2016). Therapist drift redux: Why well-meaning clinicians fail to deliver evidence-based therapy, and how to get back on track. *Behaviour Research and Therapy, 77,* 128–137.

Waller, G., Turner, H. M., Tatham, M., Mountford, V. A., & Wade, T. D. (2019). *Brief cognitive behavioural therapy for non-underweight patients: CBT-T for eating disorders.* Hove, England: Routledge.

Waller, G., Walsh, K. D. S., & Wright, C. (2016). Impact of education on clinicians' attitudes to exposure therapy for eating disorders. *Behaviour Research and Therapy, 76,* 76–80.

Wasil, A., Venturo-Conerly, K., Shingleton, R., & Weisz, J. (2019). The motivating role of recovery self-disclosures from therapists and peers in eating disorder recovery: Perspectives of recovered women. *Psychotherapy, 56,* 170–180.

Weisman, J. S., & Rodebaugh, T. L. (2018). Exposure therapy augmentation: A review and extension of techniques informed by an inhibitory learning approach. *Clinical Psychology Review, 59,* 41–51.

Westmoreland, P., Krantz, M. J., & Mehler, P. S. (2016). Medical complications of anorexia nervosa and bulimia. *The American Journal of Medicine, 129,* 30–37.

Whiteside, S. P. H., Deacon, B. J., Benito, K., & Stewart, E., (2016). Factors associated with practitioners' use of exposure therapy for childhood anxiety disorders. *Journal of Anxiety Disorders, 40,* 29–36.

Whitney, J., & Eisler, I. (2005). Theoretical and empirical models around caring for someone with an eating disorder: The reorganization of family life and inter-personal maintenance factors. *Journal of Mental Health, 14,* 575–585.

Whitney, J., Haigh, R., Weinman, J., & Treasure, J. (2007). Caring for people with eating disorders: Factors associated with psychological distress and negative caregiving appraisals in carers of people with eating disorders. *British Journal of Clinical Psychology, 46,* 413–428.

Whitney, J., Murray, J., Gavan, K., Todd, G., Whitaker, W., & Treasure, J. (2005). Experience of caring for someone with anorexia nervosa: Qualitative study. *British Journal of Psychiatry, 187,* 444–459.

Wilson, G. T., Fairburn, C. G., & Agras, W. S. (1997). Cognitive behavioral therapy for bulimia nervosa. In D. M. Garner & P. E. Garfinkel (Eds.), *Handbook of treatment for eating disorders* (pp. 67–93). New York, NY: Guilford.

Wilson, J. K., & Rapee, R. M. (2005). The interpretation of negative social events in social phobia: Changes during treatment and relationship to outcome. *Behaviour Research and Therapy, 43,* 373–389.

Winn, S., Perkins, S., Murray, J., Murphy, R., & Schmidt, U. (2004). A qualitative study of the experience of caring for a person with bulimia nervosa. Part 2: Carers' needs and experiences of services and other support. *International Journal of Eating Disorders, 36,* 269–279.

Winn, S., Perkins, S., Walwyn, R., Schmidt, U., Eisler, I., Treasure, J., . . . Yi, I. (2007). Predictors of mental health problems and negative caregiving experiences in carers of adolescents with bulimia nervosa. *International Journal of Eating Disorders, 40,* 171–178.

Zabala, M. J., Macdonald, P., & Treasure, J. (2009). Appraisal of caregiving burden, expressed emotion and psychological distress in families of people with eating disorders: A systematic review. *European Eating Disorders Review, 17,* 338–349.

Zayfert, C., & Becker, C. B. (in press). *Cognitive behavioral therapy for PTSD.* New York, NY: Guilford.

Zinbarg, R. E., Craske, M. G., & Barlow, D. H. (1993). *Therapists' guide for the mastery of your anxiety and worry.* Albany NY: Graywind.

INDEX

Tables, figures, and boxes are indicated by *t*, *f*, and *b* following the page number.

For the benefit of digital users, indexed terms that span two pages (e.g., 52–53) may, on occasion, appear on only one of those pages.

absorbing calories through skin, fear of, 171, 181–83
absorbing/blotting oil from foods, 38–40, 61
accommodation, 62, 103, 185, 186, 189
    example of, 187–88
    reducing and eliminating, 191
Agras, W. S., 133
Anderson, D. A., 167
Anderson, L. M., 167
anorexia nervosa (AN), 3, 6, 107
    body image exposure, 49, 141
    cognitive therapy techniques, 176–77
    food- and eating-based exposure, 47–48, 107
    imaginal exposure, 168
    introducing exposure to extremely malnourished patients, 67–68
    key features of, 6
    safety behaviors, 4
    transdiagnostic features of, 4
anxiety, titration of, 97–101
    intensifying exposure as needed, 98
    self-injuring patients, 100
    starting with moderately challenging situations, 98
    strategic use of avoidance/distraction/safety behaviors, 99

anxiety disorders. *See also* clinician anxiety and resistance
    age of clinician and use of exposure, 208
    comorbidity between eating disorders and, 41
    content overlap between eating disorders and, 33–40
    avoidance of distressing stimuli, 35
    functional relatedness of symptoms, 40
    preoccupation with feared outcomes, 34
    safety behaviors, 37
    emotional processing theory (habituation model), 21
    forced contact *vs.* exposure therapy, 90–91, 92
    inhibitory learning model, 25–29
    interoceptive exposure, 15
    lessons from exposure with, 29–30
    unlearning model, 20
ARFID. *See* avoidant/restrictive food intake disorder
avoidance and safety behaviors. See also names of specific behaviors
    anorexia nervosa, 4
    associated with weighing, 137
    bulimia nervosa, 4–5

avoidance and safety behaviors (*cont.*)
   CBT strategies that may serve as, 89–90, 93–94
   common, 39*t*
   content overlap between anxiety and eating disorders, 35–37
   educating patients, 68–70
   functional assessment
      example of simple avoidant/safety behavior, 59*f*
      identifying specific functional roles of avoidant/safety behaviors, 61–63
      lumping together in patient education, 68–69
   service-level issues
      patient safety behaviors, 201
      team safety behaviors, 200
   strategic use of for titrating anxiety, 99
   strengthening safety learning through removal of, 28
avoidant/restrictive food intake disorder (ARFID), 5, 107
   delivering exposure therapy in the form of hierarchies, 84–85
   eating-related fear and avoidance, 8
   feared outcomes, 34–35
   key features of, 5

baggy/loose clothing, 39*t*, 61, 62–63, 93, 94
   body image disturbance, 8–9
   body image exposure, 141, 151–52
   bulimia nervosa, 4–5
   homework, 86, 87
   interoceptive exposure, 168
Barber, J. P., 212
Baumeister, R. F., 37
Becker, C. B., 209
BED. *See* binge eating disorder
Benito, K. G., 25–26
binge eating, 7–8, 19–20, 37, 46, 65–66, 112. *See also* binge eating disorder
   "binge foods," fear of, 108–11
      creating hierarchies, 110–11
      distinguishing between doing exposure and daily life tasks, 111
      identifying feared outcomes, 108–10
      maximizing speed and diversity of change, 111
   bulimia nervosa, 4, 94
   cognitive avoidance of negative emotions, 37
   cognitive therapy techniques, 180
   conditioned cues for, 9
   cue exposure, 50–52, 121
      clinician as safety signal, 129
      conducting, 128, 129
      creating hierarchies, 128
      cue monitoring form, 127*f*, 220
      evidence of effectiveness of, 50–51
      examples of cues, 123
      extinction learning, 123–24
      identifying cues, 126, 127*f*
      patient education, 125
      timing of, 129
   delay strategies and "urge surfing," 89–90
   emotion-focused exposure, 155, 156, 160–61, 162
   food- and eating-based exposure, 110, 111
   overview of, 9
binge eating disorder (BED), 5
   emotional triggers, 155
   key features of, 5
   transdiagnostic features of, 5
Blakey, S. M., 15–16, 215
BN. *See* bulimia nervosa
body image avoidance, 4–5, 8–9, 37, 86
Body Image Avoidance Questionnaire, 150
body image disturbance, 8
body image exposure, 48–50, 141
   case example, 141
   as element of other therapies, 50
   evidence of effectiveness, 48–50
      as element of other therapies, 50
      in isolation, 49
   imaginal exposure, 149
   inappropriate and hostile feedback, 151
   in isolation, 49
   mirror exposure, 49, 50, 142–47
      choice of clinician, 148
      choice of clothing, 148

cognitive dissonance-based mirror
  exposure, 145
 combining approaches, 146
 guided mirror exposure, 144
 higher-weight patients, 148–49
 low-weight patients, 148
 non-cisgender patients, 149
 patients who overuse mirrors, 147–48
 pure mirror exposure, 143, 144
 race and ethnicity, 149
 in vivo exposure, 149
body posture adjustment, 39t, 61
body/weight checking, 7–9, 37–38, 39t, 40–41, 46, 47, 138
 body image disturbance, 8–9
 body-focused exposure, 48–49, 50
 mirror exposure, 145–46, 147–48
Boswell, J. F., 167
broken leg exception, 206
bulimia nervosa (BN), 4, 94, 107
 evidence of effectiveness of body-focused exposure, 49
 evidence of effectiveness of cue exposure, 51–52
 key features of, 4
 safety behaviors, 4–5
 transdiagnostic features of, 4–5
Byrne, S. M., 75

caloric restriction, 8, 36, 38, 39t, 40, 46, 69, 141
 anorexia nervosa, 3–4
 bulimia nervosa, 4–5
CBT. See cognitive-behavioral therapy
choking, fear of, 8, 34–35, 36, 39t, 46, 84, 102, 107–8, 117–18, 167
clinician anxiety and resistance, 205
 age of clinician, 208
 broken leg exception, 206
 colluding with patients in avoiding anxiety, 23
 institutional resistance, 207
 mental shortcuts, 207–8
 negative beliefs about exposure, 207
 reliance on clinical judgment, 205–7
 reluctance to weigh patients, 132–35
 spun glass theory of the mind, 206
 strategies for reducing
  changing clinician behaviors, 211
  changing clinician beliefs and attitudes, 209
  exposure for exposure therapists, 210
  first-hand experience, 210
  increasing clinician knowledge, 209
  supervision, 211
  treatment for anxiety disorder, 210
cognitive dissonance-based mirror exposure, 145
cognitive remediation therapy (CRT), 48
cognitive restructuring, 160, 175–77, 179–80
cognitive therapy techniques, 175, 214
 behavioral techniques vs., 175–77
 interaction effects, 175–76
 when not to use, 177–79
 when patient is extremely hesitant to engage, 181
 when predominant negative emotion is not fear, 179
cognitive-behavioral therapy (CBT), 66
 alternative activities, 89–90
 body-focused exposure as element of, 50
 cognitive strategies, 175–77
 comparison of exposure with previous therapies, 74
 cue exposure as element of, 51
 cue exposure as second-stage therapy, 52
 delay strategies and "urge surfing," 89–90
 effectiveness of, 41–42
 exposure therapy as core component of, 11, 66–67
 stimulus control strategies, 89–90
 strategies that may serve as avoidance/safety behaviors, 89–90, 93–94
 weighing patients, 131–32
comparison of self to others, 39t, 62
compulsive/excessive exercise, 4, 7–8, 19–20, 38, 39t, 42, 46, 47, 94, 95
 anorexia nervosa, 4
 fear of missing, 171

compulsive/excessive exercise (*cont.*)
   food- and eating-based exposure, 114, 115
   forced contact *vs.* exposure therapy, 91, 92
   planning exposure therapy, 77–78, 79–80, 81
conflict-averseness, 192
Contreras, I., 207
Conway, C. C., 19
Cooper, P. J., 51
Cowdrey, N. D., 66–67
Craske, M. G., 19, 25–26, 94
Crits-Christoph, P., 212
CRT (cognitive remediation therapy), 48
cue exposure
   for binge eating, 121
      clinician as safety signal, 129
      conducting, 128, 129
      creating hierarchies, 128
      cue monitoring form, 127*f*, 220
      examples of cues, 123
      extinction learning, 123–24
      identifying cues, 126, 127*f*
      patient education, 125
      timing of, 129
   evidence of effectiveness, 50–52
      controlled studies, 51
      initial studies, 51
      as second-stage therapy, 52
   theoretical underpinnings of, 122–24
   traditional exposure *vs.*, 124

D-cycloserine (DCS), 48
Deacon, B. J., 15–16, 210, 215
delay strategies, 78, 80, 89–90, 93, 111
Dennhag, I., 212
Diagnostic and Statistical Manual of Mental Disorders-Fifth Edition (DSM-5), 5, 6
dieting, 5, 7, 19–20, 69
   binge eating, 9
   binge eating disorder, 5
Dimeff, L. A., 207
distress tolerance, 93, 97–98, 100, 192
diuretic abuse. *See* laxative/diuretic abuse

Dixon, L. J., 15–16, 210
DSM-5 (*Diagnostic and Statistical Manual of Mental Disorders-Fifth Edition*), 5, 6

eating disorder not otherwise specified (EDNOS), 6
eating disorders (EDs), 11
   comorbidity between anxiety disorders and, 41
   content overlap between anxiety disorders and, 33–40
      avoidance of distressing stimuli, 35
      functional relatedness of symptoms, 40
      preoccupation with feared outcomes, 34
      safety behaviors, 37
   diagnoses, 3–6
      anorexia nervosa, 3
      avoidant/restrictive food intake disorder, 5
      binge eating disorder, 5
      bulimia nervosa, 4
      other specified feeding or eating disorder, 6
      unspecified feeding or eating disorder, 6
   feared outcomes, 34
   functional assessment, 57
      case example, 57–58
      chaining of behaviors, 60*f*
      changing pattern of behaviors, 60
      example of simple avoidant/safety behavior, 59*f*
      identifying specific functional roles of avoidant/safety behaviors, 61–63
      key lessons, 63
      methods of assessment, 61–63
      overview of, 58–60
      risk identification and management, 58
   lessons from exposure with anxiety disorders, 29–30
   rationale for applying exposure therapy to, 41–43

Index

transdiagnostic features of, 7–9
  binge eating, 9
  body image disturbance, 8
  eating-related fear and avoidance, 8
trivialization of, 3
eating-related fear and avoidance, 8, 116–18
  creating hierarchies, 118
  texture of food, 116–18
EDNOS (eating disorder not otherwise specified), 6
EDs. *See* eating disorders
educating patients. *See* patient education
emotional processing theory. *See* habituation model
emotion-focused exposure, 155–61
  addressing emotions using exposure, 159
  case example, 156
  emotions as consequence *vs.* causal factor, 155–56
  formulating role of emotions, 157
  Newton's cradle model, 157*f*, 157–59
enabling, 185, 186, 188
enemas, 57–58, 59–60
Erceg-Hurn, D. M., 75
exercise. *See* compulsive/excessive exercise
exposure therapy, 11, 89, 165. *See also* family involvement; patient education
  body image exposure, 141
  case example, 12–13
  cognitive therapy techniques for augmenting, 175
    behavioral techniques *vs.*, 176–77
    when not to use, 177–79
    when patient is extremely hesitant to engage, 181
    when predominant negative emotion is not fear, 179
  cue exposure for binge eating, 121
  decisions to make before beginning, 89
  defined, xi, 11
  development of, xi
  emotion-focused exposure, 155–61
  evidence of effectiveness, 47, 219

  body-focused exposure, 48–50
  cue exposure, 50–52
  food-based exposure, 46–48
  other exposure strategies, 52
food- and eating-based exposure, 107
forced contact *vs.*, 90–93
future directions in, 214–15
hierarchies, delivering exposure therapy in the form of, 84–85, 94–97
institutional resistance to, 195
  service-level issues, 199–202
  team dynamics, 195–98
interpersonal evaluation exposure, 161–63
key aims of, 11–12
lessons from exposure with anxiety disorders, 29–30
"lifestyle exposure," 101–2
models of, 20
  emotional processing theory (habituation model), 21–22*f*, 21
  inhibitory learning model, 25–29
  unlearning model, 20
planning, 77
  collaboration, 87
  ecological validity, 77–80
  homework, 86, 87
  learning opportunities, 80–82
  length of the session, 86–87
  "mixing it up," 84–86
  treatment settings, 82–83
positive reinforcement and praise, 81–82
present status of, 213–14
rationale for, 33
  comorbidity, 41
  content overlap, 33–40
  exposure-based nature of many evidence-based treatments, 41–43
relationship with other therapeutic strategies, 89–90, 93–94
systematic desensitization *vs.*, 25
tips for clinician improvement, 216
titrating anxiety, 97–101
  intensifying exposure as needed, 98
  self-injuring patients, 100

exposure therapy (*cont.*)
  starting with moderately challenging situations, 98
  strategic use of avoidance/distraction/safety behaviors, 99
  types of, 13–16
    imaginal exposure, 13, 168
    interoceptive exposure, 15, 165
    magical thinking exposure, 170
    virtual reality exposure, 16
    in vivo (in reality) exposure, 13
  weighing and weight exposure, 131
expressed emotion, 185, 186–87, 189
extinction learning, 41, 123–24, 125

Fairburn, C. G., 133, 147–48
family involvement, 185
  feeding for weight recovery *vs.* exposure, 193
  firm empathy, 189–90
  problematic styles of family interaction, 186–89
    accommodation, 186, 187–88, 189
    enabling, 186, 188
    expressed emotion, 186–87, 189
  psychosocial burden of EDs on family, 186
  role of family in exposure, 190–91
    family as exposure "coaches," 191
    family as exposure stimuli, 190
    reducing and eliminating accommodation, 191
family-based treatment (FBT), 41–42
Farrell, N. R., 15–16, 210, 215
fasting, 4, 7
firm empathy, 189–90, 191
flying phobia, 16
food- and eating-based exposure, 107
  evidence of effectiveness, 46–48
    case series, 47
    controlled trials, 48
    overview of, 47
    single case studies, 47
  fear of "binge foods," 108–11
    creating hierarchies, 110–11
    distinguishing between doing exposure and daily life tasks, 111
    identifying feared outcomes, 108–10
    maximizing speed and diversity of change, 111
  fear of eating, 116–18
    creating hierarchies, 118
    texture of food, 116–18
  fear of uncontrollable weight gain, 112–16
    considering biological state, 112
    considering maintaining factors, 112
    degree of voluntary engagement, 113
    graded approach, 113–16
    testing fear predictions, 113–14
  goal of, 107–8
  varying focus by profession, 107
food-related research, 37–38, 39*t*
forced contact *vs.* exposure therapy, 90–93
functional assessment, 57
  case example, 57–58
  chaining of behaviors, 60*f*
  changing pattern of behaviors, 60
  example of simple avoidant/safety behavior, 59*f*
  identifying specific functional roles of avoidant/safety behaviors, 61–63
  key lessons, 63
  methods of assessment
    direct questions, 61
    gathering information from family/friends/professionals, 62
    measures and questionnaires, 62
    observation, 62–63
    routine interview questions, 61
  overview of, 58–60
  risk identification and management, 58
Fursland, A., 75

Gallop, R., 212
generalized anxiety disorder (GAD), 14–15, 168
Gibbons, M. B. C., 212
guided mirror exposure, 144

habituation model (emotional processing theory), 21–22*f*, 21, 94–95
  between-session habituation, 21, 24–26

Index

colluding with patients in avoiding anxiety, 23
graduated exposure, 22, 23
hierarchy of fears and experiences, 21
intensive exposure (flooding), 22–23
mirror exposure, 144–45
pure mirror exposure, 143, 144–45
subjective units of distress, 22
within-session habituation, 21, 24–26
handout for patient education, 217
binge cue monitoring form, 220
evidence of effectiveness, 219
how exposure can help, 217–18
how exposure works, 218–19
Harned, M. S., 207
Heatherton, T. F., 37
hierarchies, delivering exposure therapy in the form of, 84–85, 94–97
creating hierarchies, 96, 97f
cue exposure for binge eating, 128
emotional processing theory, 21
fear of "binge foods," 110–11
fear of eating, 118
interpersonal evaluation exposure, 163
homeostasis, 122–23
homework, 86, 87

imaginal exposure, 52, 168–70, 207
body image exposure, 149
overview of, 13
utility of, 168
in vivo (in reality) exposure
body image exposure, 149
overview of, 13
inhibitory learning model, 25–29, 111, 123–24, 129, 215
clinician anxiety and resistance, 209
cognitive therapy techniques, 175–76, 177, 178–79
emotion-focused exposure, 162–63
family involvement, 193
habituation model *vs.*, 25–26
hierarchies, 94–95
imaginal exposure, 169
interoceptive exposure, 168
mirror exposure, 144–45, 146–47
"mixing it up," 84

safety learning, 26–28
service-level issues, 201–2
team dynamics, interference from, 196
weighing and weight exposure, 136, 138
institutional resistance to exposure, 195
service-level issues, 199–202
intensive care settings, 200–2
outpatient service, 199
team dynamics, 195–98
protecting patient from therapist, 196
team-based operational rules, 197
weakest link in team, 198
intensive care settings, 200–2
food- and eating-based exposure, 202
intensive care, 83
patient safety behaviors, 201
team safety behaviors, 200
interoceptive exposure, 165–68
exercises, 167
intolerance of physical sensations, 165–66
lack of clarity about physical sensations, 165–66
overview of, 15
utility of, 165
interpersonal evaluation exposure, 155, 161–63
during eating, 162
hierarchy of steps, 163

Jansen, A., 122, 123, 129

Kemp, J. J., 15–16, 215

laxative/diuretic abuse, 4, 39t, 75
length of sessions, 86–87
Levinson, C. A., 52, 168
Linehan, M. M., 68–69
loose clothing. *See* baggy/loose clothing

magical thinking exposure, 170–71
examples of, 170–71
thought-action fusion, 170
thought-shape fusion, 170
utility of, 170
manipulating food, 38–40, 39t, 92

Mavissakalian, M., 47
McEvoy, P. M., 75
medical catastrophes, fear of, 8, 34, 46
Meehl, P. E., 206, 207–8
Meyer, J. M., 207, 215
mirror exposure, 49, 50, 86, 87, 142–47
   choice of clinician, 148
   choice of clothing, 148
   cognitive dissonance-based mirror exposure, 145
   combining approaches, 146
   guided mirror exposure, 144
   higher-weight patients, 148–49
   low-weight patients, 148
   non-cisgender patients, 149
   patients who overuse mirrors, 147–48
   pure mirror exposure, 143, 144
   race and ethnicity, 149
"mixing it up," 84–86
Mountford, V. A., 36, 131
Mulkens, S., 133
Murray, S. B., 193

napkin use, 4, 38–40, 92
Newton's cradle model, 157f, 157–59

obsessive-compulsive disorder (OCD)
   accommodation, 188
   cognitive-behavioral therapy, 11
   imaginal exposure, 14, 168–69
   magical thinking, 170
   psychosocial burden on family, 186
   underutilization of exposure, 207
   in vivo (in reality) exposure, 13
odd food mixtures, 4, 38–40, 39t
other specified feeding or eating disorder (OSFED), 6
overdressing to induce sweating, 39t

panic disorder
   cognitive-behavioral therapy, 11, 177
   interoceptive exposure, 15, 166, 167
   in vivo (in reality) exposure, 13
Parker, Z. J., 207
patient education, 65

analogies, 72
asking patient how they would explain exposure to someone else, 73
comparison with other disorders, 73
comparison with previous therapies, 74
cue exposure for binge eating, 125
function of avoidance/safety behaviors, 68–70
handout, 217
   binge cue monitoring form, 220
   evidence of effectiveness, 219
   how exposure can help, 217–18
   how exposure works, 218–19
historical review of unintended exposure experiences, 73
how exposure works, 70–72
learning opportunities, 80–82
   changes can be made, 80
   feared object doesn't merit anxiety, 80
   tolerance of anxiety, 80
lumping avoidance and safety behaviors together in, 68–69
methods for, 68–75
need for, 66–67
process and mechanisms of exposure, 68
psychoeducation as exposure, 75
timing of, 67–68
Pavlovian conditioning, 122, 123
pica, 7
planning exposure therapy, 77
   collaboration, 87
   ecological validity, 77–80
   homework, 86, 87
   learning opportunities, 80–82
      changes can be made, 80
      feared object doesn't merit anxiety, 80
      tolerance of anxiety, 80
   length of the session, 86–87
   "mixing it up," 84–86
   treatment settings, 82–83
      intensive care, 83
      setting up, 82
      weighing patients, 83
posttraumatic stress disorder (PTSD)

cognitive-behavioral therapy, 11
imaginal exposure, 13–14, 169, 207
interoceptive exposure, 15–16
virtual reality exposure, 16
in vivo (in reality) exposure, 13
pure mirror exposure, 143, 144
purging behaviors, 6, 38, 42, 57–58, 60*f*, 60, 62, 180. *See also* vomiting
bulimia nervosa, 4
cue exposure, 51
emotion-focused exposure, 155–56

quick/rapid eating, 5, 7–8, 39*t*, 46

Rapp, J., 52
reassurance, seeking from others, 39*t*, 61, 62
Riley, E. N., 52
rumination disorder, 7
Raykos, B., 176–77

safety learning, 11–12, 29–30, 70, 85, 92, 93, 95, 97–98, 100, 101, 102, 169
cognitive therapy techniques, 177
defined, 68
strategies for strengthening, 26–28, 168, 193, 197–98
selective food avoidance, 36
self-injuring patients, 100
service-level issues, 199–202
intensive care settings, 200–2
food- and eating-based exposure, 202
patient safety behaviors, 201
team safety behaviors, 200
outpatient service, 199
shopping avoidance and exposure, 86
Slater, L., 206
slow eating, 4, 8, 36, 38–40, 39*t*
small bites, practice of taking, 8, 38–40, 39*t*
social anxiety disorder, 41, 142, 165
cognitive-behavioral therapy, 11
interpersonal evaluation exposure, 161–62
virtual reality exposure, 16
in vivo (in reality) exposure, 13
social mishap exposure, 13
social phobia, 15–16, 29

specific phobias
cognitive-behavioral therapy, 11
virtual reality exposure, 16
in vivo (in reality) exposure, 13
spun glass theory of the mind, 206
Steere, J., 51
Steinglass, J., 47–48
systematic desensitization, 25

team dynamics, interference from, 195–98
protecting patient from therapist, 196
team-based operational rules, 197
weakest link in team, 198
tearing/ripping food, 4, 39*t*, 47
texture-related disgust/anxiety, 34, 40, 46, 116–18
thought-action fusion, 170
thought-shape fusion, 170
Treanor, M., 19
treatment settings, 82–83
anxiety-inducing potential of, 82
intensive care, 83, 200–2
setting up, 82
waiting rooms, 82–83
weighing patients, 83

uncontrollable weight gain, fear of, 112–16
considering biological state, 112
considering maintaining factors, 112
degree of voluntary engagement, 113
graded approach, 113–16
testing fear predictions, 113–14
underdressing to induce shivering, 39*t*
unlearning model, 20
unspecified feeding or eating disorder, 6
"urge surfing," 89–90

Vervliet, B., 19
virtual reality exposure, 16, 52
Vitousek, K., 38–40, 162–63, 211
voluntary engagement in exposure therapy, 67–68, 90–91, 113
vomiting. *See also* purging behaviors
fear of, 5–6, 34, 46
self-induced, 4, 39*t*, 52, 57–58, 59–60, 62, 69

waiting rooms, 82–83
Waller, G., 36, 131, 176–77, 207
weighing and weight exposure, 83, 131
   clinician reluctance to weigh patients, 131, 132–35
   reasons for weighing patients, 131
   safety behaviors associated with weighing, 137
   strategies for, 135–38
   team-based operational rules, 197–98
weight checking. *See* body/weight checking
Wilson, G. T., 133
Woodcock, E. A., 207

Zbozinek, T., 19

www.ingramcontent.com/pod-product-compliance
Ingram Content Group UK Ltd.
Pitfield, Milton Keynes, MK11 3LW, UK
UKHW021318180426
11947UKWH00015B/1295